Back Pain

Back Pain

氣功防治腰酸背疼

- *Chinese Qigong for Healing & Prevention* -

YMAA Publication Center
Jamaica Plain, Mass. USA

YMAA Publication Center
38 Hyde Park Avenue
Jamaica Plain, Massachusetts, 02130

First Printing
5

Publisher's Cataloging in Publication
(Prepared by Quality Books Inc.)

Yang, Jwing-Ming, 1946-
    Back Pain : Chinese qigong for healing & prevention / author
Jwing-Ming Yang. — 1st ed.
    p. cm.
    Includes bibliographical references and index.
    ISBN: 1-886969-51-5

    1. Backache—Alternative treatment. 2. Backache—Prevention.
3. Ch'i kung. I. Title.

    RD771.B217Y36 1997   617.5'64
                                                QBI97-698

Figures 1-15, 1-16, 2-7, 2-12, 6-3, 6-26, 6-56, and 6-57 from the LifeART
Collection of Images ©1989-1997 by Techpool Studios, Columbus, OH.

Cover: (Frank H. Netter, M.D. The Ciba Collection of Medical Illustrations,
vol. 1, The Nervous System, Plate 9, © 1983 Novartis)

Printed in Canada.

Acknowledgments

Thanks to Tim Comrie for his photography and cover design, and Jerry Leake for his typesetting. Thanks also to Mei-Ling Yang and John Foster for general help, to Ray Ahles, Jeff Grace, Corlius Birkill, Kain Sanderson, Marc Noblitt, Andrew Murray, Jeffrey Pratt, Sean Wargo, and many other YMAA members for proofing the manuscript and for contributing many valuable suggestions and discussions. Special thanks to James O'Leary for his editing, and to Dr. Gutheil for his foreword. Thanks to Roger Whidden and Jeff Rosen for their testimonials, and to Sarah Noack for her work with the LifeART images.

ROMANIZATION OF CHINESE WORDS

YMAA Publication Center uses the Pinyin romanization system of Chinese to English. Pinyin is standard in the People's Republic of China, and in several world organizations, including the United Nations. Pinyin, which was introduced in China in the 1950's, replaces the Wade-Giles and Yale systems.

Some common conversions:

Pinyin	Also Spelled As	Pronunciation
Qi	Chi	Chee
Qigong	Chi Kung	Chee Kung
Qin Na	Chin Na	Chin Na
Jin	Jing	Jin
Gongfu	Kung Fu	Gong Foo
Taijiquan	Tai Chi Chuan	Tai Jee Chuen

For more complete conversion tables, please refer to the *People's Republic of China: Administrative Atlas*, the *Reform of the Chinese Written Language*, or a contemporary manual of style.

Contents

Chapter 1. About Chinese Qigong

Chapter 2. Understanding Our Back

Chapter 3. What are the Possible Causes of Back Pain?

Chapter 4. How Does Western Medicine Treat Back Pain?

Chapter 5. How do the Chinese Treat Back Pain?

Chapter 6. Qigong for Back Pain

Chapter 7. Conclusion

Appendix A. Translation and Glossary of Chinese Terms

Index

About the Author

Yang, Jwing-Ming, Ph.D. 楊俊敏

Dr. Yang, Jwing-Ming was born on August 11th, 1946, in Xinzhu Xian (新竹縣), Taiwan (台灣), Republic of China (中華民國). He started his Wushu (武術)(Gongfu or Kung Fu, 功夫) training at the age of fifteen under the Shaolin White Crane (Bai He, 少林白鶴) Master Cheng, Gin-Gsao (曾金灶). Master Cheng originally learned Taizuquan (太祖拳) from his grandfather when he was a child. When Master Cheng was fifteen years old, he started learning White Crane from Master Jin, Shao-Feng (金紹峰), and followed him for twenty-three years until Master Jin's death.

In thirteen years of study (1961-1974 A.D.) under Master Cheng, Dr. Yang became an expert in the White Crane Style of Chinese martial arts, which includes the use of barehands and of various weapons such as saber, staff, spear, trident, two short rods, and many other weapons. With the same master he also studied White Crane Qigong (氣功), Qin Na (or Chin Na, 擒拿), Tui Na (推拿) and Dian Xue massages (點穴按摩), and herbal treatment.

At the age of sixteen, Dr. Yang began the study of Yang Style Taijiquan (楊氏太極拳) under Master Kao Tao (高濤). After learning from Master Kao, Dr. Yang continued his study and research of Taijiquan with several masters and senior practitioners such as Master Li, Mao-Ching (李茂清) and Mr. Wilson Chen (陳威伸) in Taipei (台北). Master Li learned his Taijiquan from the well-known Master Han, Ching-Tang (韓慶堂), and Mr. Chen learned his Taijiquan from Master Chang, Xiang-San (張祥三). Dr. Yang has mastered the Taiji barehand sequence, pushing hands, the two-man fighting sequence, Taiji sword, Taiji saber, and Taiji Qigong.

When Dr. Yang was eighteen years old he entered Tamkang College (淡江學院) in Taipei Xian to study Physics. In college he began the study of traditional Shaolin Long Fist (Changquan or Chang Chuan, 少林長拳) with Master Li, Mao-Ching at the Tamkang College Guoshu Club (淡江國術社)(1964-1968 A.D.), and eventually became an assistant instructor under Master Li. In 1971 he completed his M.S. degree in Physics at the National Taiwan University (台灣大學), and then served in the Chinese Air Force from 1971 to 1972. In the service, Dr. Yang taught Physics at the Junior Academy of the Chinese Air Force (空軍幼校) while also teaching Wushu. After being honorably discharged in 1972, he returned to Tamkang College to teach Physics and resumed study under Master Li, Mao-Ching. From Master Li, Dr. Yang learned Northern Style Wushu, which includes both barehand (especially kicking) techniques and numerous weapons.

In 1974, Dr. Yang came to the United States to study Mechanical Engineering at Purdue University. At the request of a few students, Dr. Yang began to teach Gongfu (Kung Fu), which resulted in the foundation of the Purdue University Chinese Kung Fu Research Club in the spring of 1975. While at Purdue, Dr. Yang also taught college-credited courses in Taijiquan. In May of 1978 he was awarded a Ph.D. in Mechanical Engineering by Purdue.

In 1980, Dr. Yang moved to Houston to work for Texas Instruments. While in Houston he founded Yang's Shaolin Kung Fu Academy, which was eventually taken over by his disciple Mr. Jeffery Bolt after he moved to Boston in 1982. Dr. Yang founded Yang's Martial Arts Academy (YMAA) in Boston on October 1, 1982.

In January of 1984 he gave up his engineering career to devote more time to research, writing, and teaching. In March of 1986 he purchased property in the Jamaica Plain area of Boston to be used as the headquarters of the new organization, Yang's Martial Arts Association. The organization has continued to expand, and, as of July 1st 1989, YMAA has become just one division of Yang's Oriental Arts Association, Inc. (YOAA, Inc).

In summary, Dr. Yang has been involved in Chinese Wushu since 1961. During this time, he has spent thirteen years learning Shaolin White Crane (Bai He), Shaolin Long Fist (Changquan), and Taijiquan. Dr. Yang has more than twenty-eight years of instructional experience: seven years in Taiwan, five years at Purdue University, two years in Houston, Texas, and fourteen years in Boston, Massachusetts.

In addition, Dr. Yang has also been invited to offer seminars around the world to share his knowledge of Chinese martial arts and Qigong. The countries he has visited include Canada, Mexico, France, Italy, Poland, England, Ireland, Portugal, Switzerland, Germany, Hungary, Spain, Holland, Latvia, South Africa, and Saudi Arabia.

Since 1986, YMAA has become an international organization, which currently includes 30 schools located in Poland, Portugal, France, Italy, Holland, Hungary, South Africa, the United Kingdom, Canada, and the United States. Many of Dr. Yang's books and videotapes have been translated into languages such as French, Italian, Spanish, Polish, Czech, Bulgarian, Russian, and Hungarian.

Dr. Yang has published twenty-one other volumes on the martial arts and Qigong:

1. ***Shaolin Chin Na;*** Unique Publications, Inc., 1980.
2. ***Shaolin Long Fist Kung Fu;*** Unique Publications, Inc., 1981.
3. ***Yang Style Tai Chi Chuan;*** Unique Publications, Inc., 1981.
4. ***Introduction to Ancient Chinese Weapons;*** Unique Publications, Inc., 1985.
5. ***Chi Kung—Health and Martial Arts;*** YMAA Publication Center, 1985.
6. ***Northern Shaolin Sword;*** YMAA Publication Center, 1985.
7. ***Tai Chi Theory and Martial Power;*** YMAA Publication Center, 1986.
8. ***Tai Chi Chuan Martial Applications;*** YMAA Publication Center, 1986.
9. ***Analysis of Shaolin Chin Na;*** YMAA Publication Center, 1987.
10. ***Eight Simple Qigong Exercises for Health;*** YMAA Publication Center, 1988.
11. ***The Root of Chinese Qigong—Secrets for Health, Longevity, and Enlightenment;*** YMAA Publication Center, 1989.

12. ***Muscle/Tendon Changing and Marrow/Brain Washing Chi Kung—The Secret of Youth;*** YMAA Publication Center, 1989.

13. ***Hsing Yi Chuan—Theory and Applications;*** YMAA Publication Center, 1990.

14. ***The Essence of Tai Chi Chi Kung—Health and Martial Arts;*** YMAA Publication Center, 1990.

15. ***Arthritis—The Chinese Way of Healing and Prevention;*** YMAA Publication Center, 1991.

16. ***Chinese Qigong Massage—General Massage;*** YMAA Publication Center, 1992.

17. ***How to Defend Yourself;*** YMAA Publication Center, 1992.

18. ***Baguazhang—Emei Baguazhang;*** YMAA Publication Center, 1994.

19. ***Comprehensive Applications of Shaolin Chin Na—The Practical Defense of Chinese Seizing Arts;*** YMAA Publication Center, 1995.

20. ***Taiji Chin Na—The Seizing Art of Taijiquan;*** YMAA Publication Center, 1995.

21. ***The Essence of Shaolin White Crane;*** YMAA Publication Center, 1996.

Dr. Yang has also published the following videotapes:

1. ***Yang Style Tai Chi Chuan and Its Applications;*** YMAA Publication Center, 1984.

2. ***Shaolin Long Fist Kung Fu—Lien Bu Chuan and Its Applications;*** YMAA Publication Center, 1985.

3. ***Shaolin Long Fist Kung Fu—Gung Li Chuan and Its Applications;*** YMAA Publication Center, 1986.

4. ***Analysis of Shaolin Chin Na;*** YMAA Publication Center, 1987.

5. ***Eight Simple Qigong Exercises for Health—The Eight Pieces of Brocade;*** YMAA Publication Center, 1987.

6. ***Chi Kung for Tai Chi Chuan;*** YMAA Publication Center, 1990.

7. ***Arthritis—The Chinese Way of Healing and Prevention;*** YMAA Publication Center, 1991.

8. ***Qigong Massage—Self Massage;*** YMAA Publication Center, 1992.

9. ***Qigong Massage—With a Partner;*** YMAA Publication Center, 1992.

10. ***Defend Yourself 1—Unarmed Attack;*** YMAA Publication Center, 1992.

11. ***Defend Yourself 2—Knife Attack;*** YMAA Publication Center, 1992.

12. ***Comprehensive Applications of Shaolin Chin Na 1;*** YMAA Publication Center, 1995.

13. *Comprehensive Applications of Shaolin Chin Na 2;* YMAA Publication Center, 1995.

14. *Shaolin Long Fist Kung Fu—Yi Lu Mai Fu & Er Lu Mai Fu;* YMAA Publication Center, 1995.

15. *Shaolin Long Fist Kung Fu—Shi Zi Tang;* YMAA Publication Center, 1995.

16. *Taiji Chin Na;* YMAA Publication Center, 1995.

17. *Emei Baguazhang 1—Basic Training, Qigong, Eight Palms, and Applications;* YMAA Publication Center, 1995.

18. *Emei Baguazhang 2—Swimming Body Baguazhang and Its Applications;* YMAA Publication Center, 1995.

19. *Emei Baguazhang 3—Bagua Deer Hook Sword and Its Applications;* YMAA Publication Center, 1995.

20. *Xingyiquan—12 Animal Patterns and Their Applications;* YMAA Publication Center, 1995.

21. *Simplified Tai Chi Chuan—Simplified 24 Postures & Standard 48 Postures;* YMAA Publication Center, 1995.

22. *Tai Chi Chuan & Applications—Simplified 24 Postures with Applications & Standard 48 Postures;* YMAA Publication Center, 1995.

23. *White Crane Hard Qigong;* YMAA Publication Center, 1997.

24. *White Crane Soft Qigong;* YMAA Publication Center, 1997.

25. *Xiao Hu Yan—Intermediate Level Long Fist Sequence;* YMAA Publication Center, 1997

26. *Back Pain—Chinese Qigong for Healing and Prevention;* YMAA Publication Center, 1997.

27. *The Scientific Foundation of Chinese Qigong;* YMAA Publication Center, 1997.

Foreword

Ever since primitive man and woman reared up from their knuckles into the upright posture, the groan of "My aching back!" has echoed down the corridors of history in workplaces, homes, and hospitals. There are many reasons for this historical fact, a number of which have to do with life style changes, fitness, and the modern environment, all of which are spelled out by Dr. Yang in the preface to this book. Not only does the back 'carry' the body, but it also 'carries' many of the psychological tensions that constitute our modern lot.

In my psychiatric training, I learned this: to look at posture and body position for clues to a person's mental state: the stooped back whose owner seemed bowed by the weight of depression, the shoulders drawn in and tight and the head retracted like a turtle's in anticipation of a blow that comes only in the patient's imagination, and similar signs.

In my medical training I learned this: back pain is one of the hardest conditions to treat effectively. The most common approaches—protracted bed rest, lying on a firm surface, time off from work—are extremely difficult for the average person to follow. Noncompliance with the regimen is extremely common. Pain medications work somewhat, but risk addiction. Muscle relaxants work somewhat, but have troubling side effects. Surgery works as a last resort, but can make some cases worse. As a young doctor my heart would sink whenever a case of lower back pain came into the clinical emergency room, because each one carried with it the specter of the failure of Western medicine.

In my Gongfu training with Dr. Yang I learned this: he is a dedicated scholar and a gifted teacher. He merits the highest praise, however, for his efforts to meld Eastern and Western medical understanding in the hopes of achieving greater synergy between the two—that the two world views, combined, will be greater than the sum of their parts.

To this end he has written a comprehensive and wide ranging exploration of Qi theory from its historical to its present context; of the structure and function of the back; and of the Western and Eastern approaches to healing it. The first chapter alone serves as an excellent and clear introduction to the basic Eastern medical and martial arts idea of Qi. So well structured is this discussion that it requires no previous familiarity with this concept. The remainder of the book employs clear descriptions, relevant illustrations and well organized instruction to achieve the goal of providing protection and relief from back pain.

Finally, martial arts are inseparable from morality. In the present context, Dr. Yang compassionately but firmly, like a great sports coach, warns against the moral pitfalls of impatience, laziness and fear. He encourages the readers to strive to stretch their limits—carefully!—to master pain and weakness in the back. The book you hold in your hands is a noteworthy contribution to this goal.

Thomas G. Gutheil, M.D.
Associate Professor of Psychiatry,
Harvard Medical School

Testimonial

Having a healthy back, in my case, truly required committing myself to a healthy Way of Life. Central to this healthy Way of Life has been my study of martial arts for the past twenty-three years—the last six years of which I have pursued with the guidance of Master Yang.

Many of you who read this will be able to prevent or cure back problems by simple, regular practice of the movements and methods contained in this book. Some of you may need to go much deeper as I have needed to, and solve the inner mysteries that have led to your back problems. In either case, I believe all will benefit, as I have, with regular practice of these time-tested techniques.

In my life, my poor health manifested most intensely through severe, debilitating pain in my lower back. I was often completely incapacitated during my teens and early adulthood. My suffering can be traced back to a severe injury when I was six years old. I had my toes cut off of my left foot and surgically reattached. Subsequently, my functional "club" foot distorted my whole skeletal growth through my formative years. By the age of 21, I was told by prominent medical doctors that I had the "spine of a senior citizen," "I would never be a carpenter," "I would never have a job on my feet," "I would never be a gymnast," "to get a desk job," etc. From the perspective of eliminating pain, traditional medicine could offer only drugs and surgery. I did not feel I could restore my health following this path.

Fortunately, I had been training in the martial arts for three years, and I had glimpsed a ray of hope. Although the knowledge I was exposed to was only superficial relative to the knowledge Dr. Yang shares, I was on The Way. Along The Way I found adjunctive healing modalities helpful to the development of my healthy core and spinal health. Truly, Chiropractic Acupuncture, various massage forms, dietary changes, and graduate studies in Holistic Education and Counseling have been major players in my health prescription. Again central to these healing methods was my internal development, mainly due to my daily martial arts practice. For many years I was training just to avoid pain and, depending on these "alternative" therapies, to straighten me out when I erred. Gradually, as my practice moved toward health, rather than just away from illness, my dependence on external therapies for alleviation of pain virtually ceased. Now, I can use these healing tools on occasion to prevent disorder and deepen my health.

The techniques described in this book can be made central or adjunctive to your healing process. Either way, it is important to take note of those main themes of this book that are also common to traditional martial arts learning and a core part of any health prescription. Central themes to transform your injury or sickness into a healing learning event are: taking responsibility for your life, a leap of faith (not blind faith) in the healing process, an acceptance of the difficulty of life, and a full commitment to the learning/healing/life process.

If "age is the condition of the spine" (Yogic belief), then a painful spine is an old spine. It is diseased (i.e. not at ease). Regular practice of the movements described in this book in a relaxed, centered, and grounded manner will help guide you out of disease and into ease, improve the condition of your spine, bring a loving youthful bounce back to your step, and help you to understand yourself and the mysteries of life. I know this to be true.

Roger Whidden
Martial Arts Teacher
Builder, Married, Father of Three.

Testimonial

Three days before my college graduation, I had the misfortune to be a passenger in a Subaru that broad-sided a Lincoln Continental. At the hospital, the doctor asked me what I did for my scoliosis. "What scoliosis?" I asked, unsure whether it was a spine or a liver problem. "This one," he said, holding up an x-ray that looked more like a roller coaster than a spine.

Up to that point I had no problems with my back. I trained in Karate and Gongfu, and though my left side kick and right front kick wobbled when thrown, I always assumed it had something to do with laziness. In the back of my head, I had wondered why I could do a split but not touch my toes. But, like many other 22 year-olds, I moved on to other thoughts rather than resolve those.

After the accident, I spent nearly two years trying to contain a constant, severe ache. Doctors recommended nautilus and walking. Chiropractors shrugged and apologized. Two years after the accident, I returned to Tai Chi. I also got Rolfed. Now, when I practiced diligently, I could have pain free days if I didn't stress my back. The problem with this situation was that I owned an ice cream truck business. If you have never had the pleasure, let me inform you that being an ice cream truck driver, and especially, knowing other ice cream truck drivers, can really stress your back. So, I resigned myself to low-level pain.

By 1990, I was out of the ice cream truck and in an office. I practiced my form regularly and had contained my back problems. It ached when I was tired, stressed or physically active. I was prepared to live with that.

Then, in August of 1990, I stopped by the YMAA school just to take a look. From the first warm-up exercises, I saw a new path. Spine loosening and flexing is a focal point of all of the training. It takes years to begin to understand how to move the spine, how to relax the joints and the muscles in and around the spine. The process opened my eyes. Although over the years I had bored many a friend with back pain discussions (have you ever been engaged in an interesting one?), I didn't know my back. I didn't know how to move individual pieces and relax individual muscles.

The health benefits associated with learning to move this way are enormous. I am, except when I do something stupid (and I do), entirely pain free. I own a small restaurant, where I also cook. I can spend 10 hours on my feet with the fryolators gurgling and the customers screaming and go home pain free. But it is more than that. My self-image has been transformed. I no longer feel like the person who can't help move a couch. I no longer wonder whether a hike is going to cause me pain. Though people in my classes might beg to differ, I feel supple. I can move like a reed.

I am very grateful for my YMAA training, particularly for the relaxation of my spine. It has freed me from pain, and shown me a path to healthy feeling.

Jeff Rosen

Preface

Our life style has changed in the last fifty years from the way it had endured for over a million years. Now, we sleep late, have less laborious work, walk very little, carry fewer children in a family, spend more time watching television and looking at a computer screen, more radiation passes through our body, etc. Our bodies, in a short period of time, cannot adjust themselves to fit into these new, rapidly developing life styles. Consequently, many problems occur. We are experiencing more knee pain and weakness, back degeneration and disease, breast cancer, and many other illnesses.

Today, back pain is considered by many to be one of the most serious health problems affecting our quality of life. In fact, lower back pain is the second most common cause of pain, surpassed only by headaches, and is second to the common cold as a reason for doctor's office visits in the United States. It is estimated that 31 million Americans experience back pain, at an annual cost of $16 to $20 billion in medical treatments and disability payments. The reason that there are more back pain cases today than before is simply because we now use more machinery to replace our daily muscular work. Our torso has become significantly weakened.

Therefore, if a person is not aware of the problems generated by our new life style, and fails to keep their torso healthy and fit, he or she will most likely experience back pain before their 40th birthday. The key to maintaining the health of our torso is very simple: **exercise correctly and stick with it**. Consistent exercise will slow down the aging and degeneration of the spine and build up stronger torso muscles to support your body. This is the most basic and important key to preventing back problems.

I have learned martial Qigong since the age of fifteen. From the last thirty-five years of my experience practicing and teaching, I have discovered that, among all the Qigong I have learned, the spinal Qigong exercises and meditation from the White Crane and Taijiquan styles can heal spine problems and rebuild the strength of the torso. White Crane is considered to be a soft-hard martial style, while Taijiquan is considered a soft style. In these two styles, the spine and chest are considered two major **bows,** which can generate great martial power. In order to have this power, the condition of the spine and chest is extremely important. You must learn how to move them softly, like a silken whip, while coordinating the movements with your concentrated mind and breath. You must also know how to tense the torso, so that when the power reaches the target, your spine is not injured.

In these martial arts, through hundred years of practice, spine injury sometimes occurred due to the heavy training. Therefore, self healing and conditioning of the spine has always been an essential practice in White Crane and Taijiquan.

Since 1986, I have conducted seminars in many countries and have taught these spinal Qigong techniques for health purposes. The original purpose was only to help many of the Karate practitioners in France to regain their spinal health, which they had injured through Karate practice. Later, I realized that these lower back problems were very common in Karate society, due to the strenuous Karate training. After many years of teaching, countless people have told me how they have benefited from these simple spinal Qigong exercises. I now realize that this Qigong can not only heal and rebuild the spine, but can also heal asthma, stomach problems, kidney irregularities, and most importantly of all, strengthen the body's immune system.

All of these Qigong exercises were ignored by me between 1974 to 1984. During these ten years, I was busy studying for my doctorate degree and working as an engineer. It was not until late 1983 when I developed a kidney stone that I realized I was out of shape. When the doctor told me that I would most likely experience a recurrence of the kidney stone every six months, I was very frightened because of the intense pain involved. I decided to quit my engineering job, and I did on January 1, 1984. I then resumed my White Crane spinal Qigong practice and started to move the torso muscles above the kidneys. In Chinese Qigong, to tense and relax these two muscles on the kidneys is known as a kidney massage, and through correct spinal movement, the Qi and the blood circulation in the kidneys can be made smooth. Amazingly, since then, I have never experienced another kidney stone.

This book is written to share my experience with those who need to heal their spine and rebuild its strength. I deeply believe that anyone, as long as they are patient and consistent in their Qigong exercises, will see positive results within three months. Naturally, this is not an easy task. It is a challenge to your health, happiness, and joy of life.

In this book, in order to help build a theoretical foundation, I will introduce the main concepts of Qigong in chapter 1. Next, In chapter 2 we will study the structure of our back, both physically and from the Chinese Qi concepts. In chapter 3, the possible causes of back pain will be discussed. Chapter 4 will review treatments by Western doctors, and chapter 5 will summarize possible treatments of back pain by Chinese physicians. Finally, Qigong exercises for back pain and rehabilitation will be introduced in chapter 6. In this chapter, some Qigong massage techniques will be discussed and acupressure cavities will also be introduced.

CHAPTER 1

About Chinese Qigong

中國氣功介紹

1-1. Introduction

According to recent medical reports, today it is estimated that at least thirty-one million Americans experience back pain, at an annual cost of $16 to $20 billion in medical treatments and disability payments. This does not even include lost working days, which results in financial losses in both business and industry. However, the most important loss is the patient's happiness and joy of life. It is estimated that between 80-90 percent of the occurrences of lower back pain require approximately six to eight weeks of recovery time. However, once your spine is injured, it is four times more likely to get hurt again.[1]

It is believed that the majority of adults—80 percent or more—will experience at least one significant episode of lower back pain at some point in their lives. It affects men and women alike, usually occurring between the late twenties and the fifties, the middle working years of life. As is now known, lower back pain is the second most common cause of pain next to headaches, and is second only to the common cold as a reason for office visits to primary care physicians in the United States.[2]

From the above, you can see that back pain has become a serious problem for the human race. In order to solve this problem, instead of merely looking for a cure, we must also examine its causes. If we calm down and ponder carefully, we can perhaps more easily see that the main problem originates from our modern life style rather than any physiological cause. If we look at our life style, we see that laborious work has been significantly reduced and replaced by machinery. Because of this, our physical body, which has evolved for millions of years, has started to degenerate and weaken quickly. We are not in the same shape as we were a century ago.

In order to remedy this problem and prevent further loss of our back strength, first we must study our old life styles, which evolved over time to ensure our survival. No matter what, we will always be a part of nature, and we must follow the "natural way" (i.e., Dao, 道). Chinese Qigong was developed by following this Dao, through observation of the relationships between nature and humanity. It is a human historical science, and has a firm and solid theoretical and empirical foundation. Qigong concepts were not accepted by Westerners until the early 1970's, when the usefulness of acupuncture could no longer be denied. Now, more and more traditional Chinese healing techniques are being "discovered" by the west.

The most fundamental principle of Chinese medicine is the concept of Qi (氣 , pronounced 'Chee'—known today in the West as bioelectricity). Illnesses are diagnosed by evaluating the condition of the body's Qi and interpreting the visible physical symptoms. According to Chinese medicine, when the need for Qi and its supply in the body start to become unbalanced, the physical body is affected and begins to be damaged. This can happen both if the body is too Yin (deficient in Qi) or too Yang (with an excess of Qi). When Chinese physicians diagnose any disease or condition, they explore how and where the Qi is unbalanced. Once the Qi imbalance is corrected and the Qi returned to its normal level, the root cause of the illness has been removed. Acupuncture is a common method for adjusting the Qi and preventing further physical damage. The Qi level can also be raised or lowered to stimulate the repair of the damage.

While Western medicine has developed according to the principle of diagnosing visible symptoms and curing visible physical damage, Chinese medicine may be more advanced in that it deals with the body's Qi. On the other hand, Chinese medicine is still far behind Western medicine in the study and research of the physical aspects of the human body. This can be seen in Western scientific methods and in the technology the West has developed. Because of the differences between the two systems of medicine, there are still large gaps in our understanding of the body. I believe that if both medical cultures can learn and borrow from each other, these remaining gaps can soon be filled, and medicine as a whole will be able to take a giant step forward.

The ease of communication and the increased friendship among the different cultures in the last two decades has given humankind an unprecedented opportunity to share such things as medical concepts. We should all take advantage of this and open our minds to the knowledge and experiences of other peoples. I sincerely hope that this takes place, especially in the field of medicine. This goal has been my motivation in writing this book. Because of my limited knowledge, I can only offer this little volume. I hope that it generates widening ripples of interest in sharing and exchanging information with other cultures.

The first step to understanding Qigong is to know the concepts and definitions of Qi and Qigong and their relationship to humans. Therefore, we will discuss this subject in the next section. In addition, in order to trace the root of Qigong development, we will summarize a brief Qigong history and different categories which have developed in sections 3 and 4 of this chapter. Moreover, in order to provide you with a basic theoretical foundation for Qigong practice, Qigong training theory will be discussed in section 5. Finally, some keys for using this book will be listed in the last section.

1-2. Qi, Qigong, and Man

Before we discuss the relationship of Qi to the human body, we should first define Qi and Qigong. We will first discuss the general concept of Qi, including both the traditional understanding and the possible modern scientific paradigms, which allows us to use modern concepts to explain Qigong. If you would like to investigate these subjects in more detail, please refer to the YMAA book *The Root of Chinese Qigong*.

A General Definition of Qi

Qi is the energy or natural force which fills the universe. The Chinese have traditionally believed that there are three major powers in the universe. These Three Powers (San Cai, 三才) are Heaven (Tian, 天), Earth (Di, 地), and Man (Ren, 人). Heaven (the sky or universe) has Heaven Qi (Tian Qi), the most important of the three, which is made up of the forces which the heavenly bodies exert on the earth, such as sunshine, moonlight, gravity, and the energy from the stars. In ancient times, the Chinese believed that weather, climate, and natural disasters were governed by Heaven Qi. Chinese people still refer to the weather as Heaven Qi (Tian Qi, 天氣). Every energy field strives to stay in balance, so whenever the Heaven Qi loses its balance, it tries to rebalance itself. Then the wind must blow, rain must fall, even tornadoes or hurricanes must happen in order for the Heaven Qi to reach a new energy balance.

Under Heaven Qi, is Earth Qi (Di Qi, 地氣). It is influenced and controlled by Heaven Qi. For example, too much rain will force a river to flood or change its path. Without rain, the plants will die. The Chinese believe that Earth Qi is made up of lines and patterns of energy, as well as the earth's magnetic field and the heat concealed underground. These energies must also balance, otherwise disasters such as earthquakes will occur. When the Qi of the earth is balanced, plants will grow and animals thrive.

Finally, within the Earth Qi, each individual person, animal, and plant has its own Qi field, which always seeks to be balanced. When any individual thing loses its Qi balance, it will sicken, die, and decompose. All natural things, including humankind and our Human Qi, grow within and are influenced by the natural cycles of Heaven Qi and Earth Qi. Throughout the history of Qigong, people have been most interested in Human Qi and its relationship with Heaven Qi and Earth Qi.

In China, **Qi is defined as any type of energy that is able to demonstrate power and strength**. This energy can be electricity, magnetism, heat, or light. For example, electric power is called "electric Qi" (Dian Qi, 電氣), and heat is called "heat Qi" (Re Qi, 熱氣). When a person is alive, his body's energy is called "human Qi" (Ren Qi, 人氣).

Qi is also commonly used to express the energy state of something, especially living things. As mentioned before, the weather is called "Heaven Qi" (Tian Qi, 天氣) because it indicates the energy state of the heavens. When something is alive it has "vital Qi" (Huo Qi, 活氣), and when it is dead it has "dead Qi" (Si Qi, 死氣) or "ghost Qi" (Gui Qi, 鬼氣). When a person is righteous and has the spiritual strength to do good, he is said to have "Normal Qi or Righteous Qi" (Zheng Qi, 正氣). The spiritual state or morale of an army is called "energy state" (Qi Shi, 氣勢).

You can see that the word "Qi" has a wider and more general definition than most people think. It does not refer only to the energy circulating in the human body. Furthermore, the word "Qi" can represent energy itself, and it can even be used to express the manner or state of the energy. It is important to understand this when you practice Qigong, so that your mind is not channeled into a narrow understanding of Qi, which would limit your future understanding and development.

A Narrow Definition of Qi

Now that you understand the general definition of Qi, let us look at how Qi is defined in Qigong society today. As mentioned before, among the Three Powers, the Chinese have been most concerned with the Qi which is related to our health and longevity. Therefore, after four thousand years of emphasizing Human Qi, when people mention Qi they usually mean the Qi circulating in our bodies.

If we look at the Chinese medical and Qigong documents that were written about two thousand years ago, the word "Qi" was written as 炁. This character is constructed of two words; 旡 on the top, which means "nothing;" and 灬 on the bottom, which means "fire." This means that the word "Qi" was actually written as "no fire" in ancient times. If we go back through Chinese medical and Qigong history, it is not hard to understand this expression.

In ancient times, **the Chinese physicians or Qigong practitioners were actually looking for the Yin-Yang balance of the Qi circulating in the body. When this goal was reached, there was "no fire" in the internal organs**. This concept is very simple. According to Chinese medicine, each of our internal organs needs to receive a specific amount of Qi to function properly. If an organ receives an improper amount of Qi (usually too much, i.e., too Yang), it will start to malfunction, and, in time, physical damage will occur. Therefore, the goal of the medical or Qigong practitioner was to attain a state of "no fire," which eventually became the word "Qi."

However, in more recent publications, the Qi of "no fire" has been replaced by the character 氣, which is again constructed of two characters, 气 which means "air," and 米 which means "rice." This shows that later practitioners realized that the Qi circulating in our bodies is produced mainly by the breathing of air and the consumption of food (rice). Air is called Kong Qi (空氣), which means literally "space energy."

For a long time, people were confused about just what type of energy was circulating in our bodies. Many people believed that it was heat, others considered it to be electricity, and many others assumed that it was a mixture of heat, electricity, and light.

This confusion lasted until the early 1980's, when the concept of Qi gradually became clear. If we think carefully about what we know from science, we can see that (except possibly for gravity) there is actually only one type of energy in this universe, and that is electromagnetic energy. This means that light (electromagnetic waves) and heat (infrared waves) are also part of electromagnetic energy. This makes it very clear that the Qi circulating in our bodies is actually "bioelectricity," and that our body is a "living electromagnetic field."[3&4] This field is affected by our thoughts, feelings, activities, the food we eat, the quality of the air we breathe, our life style, the natural energy that surrounds us, and also the unnatural energy which modern science inflicts upon us.

Next, let us define Qigong. Once you understand what Qigong is, you will be able to better understand the role Qigong plays in Chinese medical science.

A General Definition of Qigong

We have explained that Qi is energy, and that it is found in the heavens, in the earth, and in every living thing. The word "Gong" (功) is often used instead of "Gongfu" (or Kung Fu, 功夫), which means energy and time. Any study or training which requires a lot of energy and time to learn or to accomplish is called Gongfu. The term can be applied to any special skill or study as long as it requires time, energy, and patience. Therefore, **the correct definition of Qigong is any training or study dealing with Qi which takes a long time and a lot of effort**. You can see from this definition that Qigong is a science which studies the energy in nature. The main difference between this energy science and Western energy science is that Qigong focuses on the inner energy of human beings, while Western energy science pays more attention to the energy outside of the human body. When you study Qigong, it is worthwhile to also consider the modern, scientific point of view, and not restrict yourself to only the traditional beliefs.

The Chinese have studied Qi for thousands of years. Some of the information on the patterns and cycles of nature has been recorded in books, one of which is the *Yi Jing* (易經)(*Book of Changes;* 1122 B.C.). When the *Yi Jing* was written, the Chinese people, as mentioned earlier, believed that natural power included Heaven (Tian, 天), Earth (Di, 地), and Man (Ren, 人). These are called "The Three Powers" (San Cai, 三才) and are manifested by the three Qi's: Heaven Qi, Earth Qi, and Human Qi. These three facets of nature have their definite rules and cycles. The rules never change, and the cycles repeat regularly. The Chinese people used an understanding of these natural principles and the *Yi Jing* to calculate the changes of natural Qi. This calculation is called "The Eight Trigrams" (Bagua, 八卦). From the Eight Trigrams are derived the sixty-four hexagrams. Therefore, the *Yi Jing* was probably the first book which taught the Chinese people about Qi and its variations in nature and man. The relationship of the Three Natural Powers and their Qi variations were later discussed extensively in the book *Theory of Qi's Variation (Qi Hua Lun, 氣化論)*.

Understanding Heaven Qi is very difficult, and it was especially so in ancient times when the science was just developing. But since nature is always repeating itself, the experiences accumulated over the years have made it possible to trace the natural patterns. Understanding the rules and cycles of "heavenly timing" (Tian Shi, 天時) will help you to understand natural changes of the seasons, climate, weather, rain, snow, drought, and all other natural occurrences. If you observe carefully, you will be able to see many of these routine patterns and cycles caused by the rebalancing of the Qi fields. Among the natural cycles are those which repeat every day, month, or year, as well as cycles of twelve years and sixty years.

Earth Qi is a part of Heaven Qi. If you can understand the rules and the structure of the earth, you will be able to understand how mountains and rivers are formed, how plants grow, how rivers move, what part of the country is best for someone, where to build a house and which direction it should face so that it is a healthy place to live, and many other things related to the earth. In China today there are people, called "geomancy teachers" (Di Li Shi, 地理師) or "wind water teachers" (Feng Shui Shi, 風水師), who make their living this way. The term "wind water" (Feng Shui, 風水) is commonly used because the location and character of the wind and water in a landscape are the most important factors in evaluating a location. These experts use the accumulated body of geomantic knowledge and the *Yi Jing* to help people make important decisions such as where and how to build a house, where to bury their dead, and how to rearrange or redecorate homes and offices so that they are better places in which to live and work. Many people even believe that setting up a store or business according to the guidance of Feng Shui can make it more prosperous.

Among the three Qi's, Human Qi is probably the one studied most thoroughly. The study of Human Qi covers a large number of different subjects. The Chinese people believe that Human Qi is affected and controlled by Heaven Qi and Earth Qi, and that they in fact determine your destiny. Therefore, if you understand the relationship between nature and people, in addition to understanding "human relations" (Ren Shi, 人事), you will be able to predict wars, the destiny of a country, a person's desires and temperament, and even their future. The people who practice this profession are called "calculate life teachers" (Suan Ming Shi, 算命師).

However, the greatest achievement in the study of Human Qi is with regard to health and longevity. Since Qi is the source of life, if you understand how Qi functions and know how to regulate it correctly, you should be able to live a long and healthy life. Remember that you are part of nature, and you are channeled into the cycles of nature. If you go against this natural cycle, you may become sick, so it is in your best interest to follow the way of nature. This is the meaning of **Dao** (道) which can be translated as **"The Natural Way."**

Many different aspects of Human Qi have been researched, including acupuncture, acupressure, massage, herbal treatment, meditation, and Qigong exercises. The use of acupuncture, acupressure, and herbal treatment to adjust Human Qi flow has become the root of Chinese medical science. Meditation and moving Qigong exercises are used widely by the Chinese people to improve their health or even to cure certain illnesses. In addition, Daoists and Buddhists use meditation and Qigong exercises in their pursuit of enlightenment and Buddhahood.

In conclusion, **the study of any of the aspects of Qi including Heaven Qi, Earth Qi, and Human Qi should be called Qigong**. However, since the term is usually used today only in reference to the cultivation of Human Qi through meditation and exercises, we will only use it in this narrower sense to avoid confusion.

A Narrow Definition of Qigong

As mentioned earlier, the narrow definition of Qi is "the energy circulating in the human body." Therefore, **the narrow definition of Qigong is "the study of the Qi circulating in the human body."** Because our bodies are part of nature, the narrow definition of Qigong should also include the study of how our bodies relate to Heaven Qi and Earth Qi. Chinese Qigong today consists of several different fields: acupuncture, herbs for regulating human Qi, martial arts Qigong, Qigong massage, Qigong exercises, Qigong healing, and religious enlightenment Qigong. Naturally, these fields are mutually related, and in many cases cannot be separated.

The Chinese have discovered that the human body has twelve major Qi channels (Shi Er Jing, 十二經) and eight vessels (Ba Mai, 八脈) through which the Qi circulates. The twelve channels are like **rivers** which distribute Qi throughout the body, and also connect the extremities (fingers and toes) to the internal organs. Here you should understand that the "internal organs" of Chinese medicine do not necessarily correspond to the physical organs as understood in the West, but rather to a set of clinical functions similar to each other, and related to the organ system. The eight vessels, which are often referred to as the extraordinary vessels, function like **reservoirs** and regulate the distribution and circulation of Qi in your body.

When the Qi in the eight reservoirs is full and strong, the Qi in the rivers is strong and will be regulated efficiently. When there is stagnation in any of these twelve channels or rivers, the Qi which flows to the body's extremities and to the internal organs will be abnormal, and illness may develop. You should understand that every channel has its particular Qi flow strength, and every channel is different. All of these different levels of Qi strength are affected by your mind, the weather, the time of day, the food you have eaten, and even your mood. For example, when the weather is dry the Qi in the lungs will tend to be more positive than when it is moist. When you are angry, the Qi flow in your liver channel will be abnormal. The Qi strength in the different channels varies throughout the day in a regular cycle, and at any particular time one channel is strongest. For example, between 11 a.m. and 1 p.m. the Qi flow in the Heart Channel is the strongest. Furthermore, the Qi level of the same organ can be different from one person to another.

Whenever the Qi flow in the twelve rivers or channels is not normal, the eight reservoirs will regulate the Qi flow and bring it back to normal. For example, when you experience a sudden shock, the Qi flow in the bladder immediately becomes deficient. Normally, the reservoir will immediately regulate the Qi in this channel so that you recover from the shock. However, if the reservoir Qi is also deficient, or if the effect of the shock is too great and there is not enough time to regulate the Qi, the bladder will suddenly contract, causing unavoidable urination.

When a person is sick, his Qi level tends to be either too positive (excessive; Yang, 陽) or too negative (deficient; Yin, 陰). A Chinese physician would either use a prescription of herbs to adjust the Qi, or else he would insert acupuncture needles at various spots on the channels to inhibit the flow in some channels and stimulate the flow in others, so that balance could be restored. However, there is another alternative, and that is to use certain physical and mental exercises to adjust the Qi. In other words, to use Qigong.

The above discussion is only to offer an idea of the narrow definition of Qigong. In fact, when people talk about Qigong today, most of the time they are referring to the mental and physical exercises that work with the Qi.

A Modern Definition of Qi

It is important that you know about the progress that has been made by modern science in the study of Qi. This will keep you from getting stuck in the ancient concepts and level of understanding.

In ancient China, people had very little knowledge of electricity. They only knew from acupuncture that when a needle was inserted into the acupuncture cavities, some kind of energy other than heat was produced which often caused a shock or a tickling sensation. It was not until the last few decades, when the Chinese people were more acquainted with electromagnetic science, that they began to recognize that this energy circulating in the body, which they called Qi, might be the same thing as what today's science calls "bioelectricity."

It is understood now that the human body is constructed of many different electrically conductive materials, and that it forms a living electromagnetic field and circuit. Electromagnetic energy is continuously being generated in the human body through the biochemical reaction in food and air assimilation, and circulated by the electromotive forces (EMF) generated within the body.

In addition, you are constantly being affected by external electromagnetic fields such as that of the earth, or the electrical fields generated by clouds. When you practice Chinese medicine or Qigong, you need to be aware of these outside factors and take them into account.

Countless experiments have been conducted in China, Japan, and other countries to study how external magnetic or electrical fields can affect and adjust the body's Qi field. Many acupuncturists use magnets and electricity in their treatments. They attach a magnet to the skin over a cavity and leave it there for a period of time. The magnetic field gradually affects the Qi circulation in that channel. Alternatively, they insert needles into cavities and then run an electric current through the needle to reach the Qi channels directly. Although many researchers have claimed a degree of success in their experiments, none has been able to publish any detailed and convincing proof of the results, or give a good explanation of the theory behind the experiment. As with many other attempts to explain the How and Why of acupuncture, conclusive proof is elusive, and many unanswered questions remain. Of course, this theory is quite new, and it will probably take more study and research before it is verified and completely understood. At present, there are many conservative acupuncturists who are skeptical.

To untie this knot, we must look at what modern Western science has discovered about bioelectromagnetic energy. Many bioelectricity related reports have been published, and frequently the results are closely related to what is experienced in

Chinese Qigong training and medical science. For example, during the electrophysiological research of the 1960's, several investigators discovered that bones are piezoelectric; that is, when they are stressed, mechanical energy is converted to electrical energy in the form of electric current.[3] This might explain one of the practices of Marrow Washing Qigong in which the stress on the bones and muscles is increased in certain ways to increase the Qi circulation.

Dr. Robert O. Becker has done important work in this field. His book *The Body Electric* [4] reports on much of the research concerning the body's electric field. It is presently believed that food and air are the fuels which generate the electricity in the body through biochemical reaction. This electricity, which is circulated throughout the entire body by means of electrically conductive tissue, is one of the main energy sources that keeps the cells of the physical body alive.

Whenever you have an injury or are sick, your body's electrical circulation is affected. If this circulation of electricity stops, you die. But bioelectric energy not only maintains life, it is also responsible for repairing physical damage. Many researchers have sought ways of using external electrical or magnetic fields to speed up the body's recovery from physical injury. Richard Leviton reports: "Researchers at Loma Linda University's School of medicine in California have found, following studies in sixteen countries with over 1,000 patients, that low-frequency, low-intensity magnetic energy has been successful in treating chronic pain related to tissue ischemia, and has also worked in clearing up slow-healing ulcers, and in 90 percent of patients tested, raised blood flow significantly."[5]

Mr. Leviton also reports that every cell of the body functions like an electric battery and is able to store electric charges. He reports that: "Other biomagnetic investigators take an even closer look to find out what is happening, right down to the level of the blood, the organs, and the individual cell, which they regard as 'a small electric battery'."[5] This has convinced me that our entire body is essentially a big battery which is assembled from millions of small batteries. All of these batteries together form the human electromagnetic field.

Furthermore, much of the research on the body's electrical field relates to acupuncture. For example, Dr. Becker reports that the conductivity of the skin is much higher at acupuncture cavities, and that it is now possible to locate them precisely by measuring the skin's conductivity (Figure 1-1).[4] Many of these reports prove that the acupuncture which has been done in China for thousands of years is reasonable and scientific.

Some researchers use the theory of the body's electricity to explain many of the ancient "miracles" which have been attributed to the practice of Qigong. A report by Albert L. Huebner states: "These demonstrations of body electricity in human beings may also offer a new explanation of an ancient healing practice. If weak external fields can produce powerful physiological effects, it may be that fields from human tissues in one person are capable of producing clinical improvements in another. In short, the method of healing known as the laying on of hands could be an especially subtle form of electrical stimulation."[3]

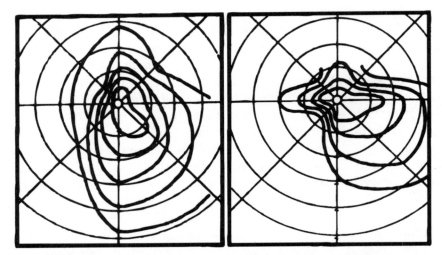

Figure 1-1. Electrical Conductivity Maps of the Skin Surface over Acupuncture Points

Another frequently reported phenomenon is that when a Qigong practitioner has reached a high level of development, a corona or halo would appear behind and/or around his head during meditation. This is commonly seen in paintings of Jesus Christ, the Buddha, and various Oriental immortals. Frequently the light is pictured as surrounding the whole body. This phenomenon may again be explained by the body electric theory. When a person has cultivated their Qi (electricity) to a high level, the Qi may be led to accumulate in the head. This Qi may then interact with the oxygen molecules in the air, and ionize them, causing them to glow.

Although the link between the theory of *The Body Electric* and the Chinese theory of Qi is becoming more accepted and better proven, there are still many questions to be answered. For example, how can the mind lead Qi (electricity)? How actually does the mind generate an EMF (electromotive force) to circulate the electricity in the body? How is the human electromagnetic field affected by the multitude of other electric fields which surround us, such as radio wiring or electrical appliances? How can we readjust our electromagnetic fields and survive in outer space or on other planets where the magnetic field is completely different from Earth's? You can see that the future of Qigong and bioelectric science is a challenging and exciting one. It is about time that we started to use modern technology to understand the inner energy world which has been for the most part ignored by Western society.

A Modern Definition of Qigong

If you now accept that the inner energy (Qi) circulating in our bodies is bioelectricity, then we can now formulate a definition of Qigong based on electrical principles.

Let us assume that the circuit shown in Figure 1-2 is similar to the circuit in our bodies. Unfortunately, although we now have a certain degree of understanding of this circuit from acupuncture, we still do not know in detail exactly what the body's circuit looks like. We know that there are twelve primary Qi channels (Qi rivers) and

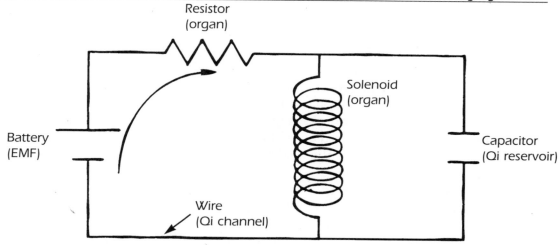

Resistor
(organ)

Solenoid
(organ)

Battery
(EMF)

Capacitor
(Qi reservoir)

Wire
(Qi channel)

Figure 1-2. The Human Bioelectric Circuit is Similar to an Electric Circuit

eight vessels (Qi reservoirs) in our body. There are also thousands of small Qi channels (Luo, 絡) which allow the Qi to reach the skin and the bone marrow. In this circuit, the twelve internal organs are connected and mutually related through these
channels.

If you look at the electrical circuit in the illustration, you will see that:

1. The Qi channels are like the wires which carry electric current.

2. The internal organs are like the electrical components such as resistors and
   solenoids.

3. The Qi vessels are like capacitors (i.e., regulators), which regulate the current in the circuit.

How do you keep this electrical circuit functioning most efficiently? Your first
concern is the resistance of the wire which carries the current. In a machine, you
want to use a wire which has a high level of conductivity and low resistance, otherwise the current may melt the wire. Therefore, the wire should be of a material like
copper or perhaps even gold. In your body, you want to keep the current flowing
smoothly. This means that your first task is to remove anything which interferes
with the flow and causes stagnation. Fat has low conductivity, so you should use diet
and exercise to remove excess fat from your body. You should also learn how to
relax your physical body, because this opens all of the Qi channels. This is why relaxation is the first goal in Taijiquan and many Qigong exercises.

Your next concern in maintaining a healthy electrical circuit is the amount of current going through the components—your internal organs. If you do not have the
correct level of current in your organs, they will either burn out from too much current (Yang) or malfunction because of a deficient level of current (Yin). In order to
avoid these problems in a machine, you use a capacitor to regulate the current.
Whenever there is too much current, the capacitor absorbs and stores the excess,
and whenever the current is weak, the capacitor supplies current to raise the level.

The eight Qi vessels are your body's capacitors. Qigong is concerned with learning how to increase the level of Qi in these vessels so that they will be able to supply current when needed, and keep the internal organs functioning smoothly. This is especially important as you get older and your Qi level is generally lower.

Finally, in order to have a healthy circuit, you have to be concerned with the components themselves. If any of them are not strong and of good quality, the entire circuit will have problems. This means that the final concern in Qigong practice is how to maintain or even rebuild the health of your internal organs. Before we go any further, we should point out that there is an important difference between the circuit shown in the diagram and the Qi circuit in our bodies. This difference is that the human body is alive, and with the proper Qi nourishment, all of the cells can be regrown and the state of health improved. For example, if you can jog about three miles today, and if you keep jogging regularly and gradually increase the distance, eventually you will be able to easily jog five miles. This is because your body rebuilds and readjusts itself to fit the circumstances.

This means that, if we can increase the Qi flow through our internal organs, they can become stronger and healthier. Naturally, the increase in Qi must be slow and gradual so that the organs can adjust to it. In order to increase the Qi flow in your body, you need to work with the EMF (electromotive force) in your body. If you do not know what EMF is, imagine two containers filled with water and connected by a tube. If both containers have the same water level, then the water will not flow. However, if one side is higher than the other, the water will flow from that container to the other. In electricity, this potential difference is called electromotive force. Naturally, the higher the EMF is, the stronger the current will flow.

You can see from this discussion that the key to effective Qigong practice is, in addition to removing resistance from the Qi channels, learning how to increase the EMF in your body. Now let us see what the sources of EMF in the body are, so that we may use them to increase the flow of bioelectricity. Generally speaking, there are five major sources:

1. **Natural Energy.** Since your body is constructed of electrically conductive material, its electromagnetic field is always affected by the sun, the moon, clouds, the earth's magnetic field, and by the other energies around you. The major influences are the sun's radiation, the moon's gravity, and the earth's magnetic field. These affect your Qi circulation significantly, and are responsible for the pattern of your Qi circulation since you were formed. We are now also being greatly affected by the energy generated by modern technology, such as the electromagnetic waves generated by radio, TV, microwave ovens, computers, and many other things.

2. **Food and Air.** In order to maintain life, we take in food and air essence through our mouth and nose. These essences are then converted into Qi through biochemical reaction in the chest and digestive system (called the Triple Burner in Chinese medicine). When Qi is converted from the essence, an EMF is generated which circulates the Qi throughout the body.

Consequently a major part of Qigong is devoted to getting the proper kinds of food and fresh air.

3. **Thinking.** The human mind is the most important and efficient source of bio-electric EMF. Any time you move to do something you must first generate an idea (Yi). This idea generates the EMF and leads the Qi to energize the appropriate muscles to carry out the desired motion. The more you can concentrate, the stronger the EMF you can generate, and the stronger the flow of Qi you can lead. Naturally, the stronger the flow of Qi you lead to the muscles, the more they will be energized. Because of this, the mind is considered the most important factor in Qigong training.

4. **Exercise.** Exercise converts the food essence (fat) stored in your body into Qi, and therefore builds up the EMF. Many Qigong styles have been created which utilize movement for this purpose. Furthermore, when you exercise, you are also using your mind to manage your physical body, and this enhances the EMF for the Qi's circulation.

5. **Converting Pre-Birth Essence into Qi.** The hormones produced by our endocrine glands are referred to as "Pre-Birth essence" in Chinese medicine. They can be converted into Qi to stimulate the functioning of our physical body, thereby increasing our vitality. Balancing hormone production when you are young and increasing its production when you are old are important subjects in Chinese Qigong.

From the above, you can see that within the human body, there is a network of electrical circuitry. In order to maintain the circulation of bioelectricity, there must be a battery wherein to store a charge. Where then, is the battery in our body?

Chinese Qigong practitioners believe that there is a place which is able to store Qi (bioelectricity). This place is called the Dan Tian (i.e., elixir field). According to such practitioners, there are three Dan Tians in the human body. One is located at the abdominal area, one or two inches below the navel, called the "Lower Dan Tian" (Xia Dan Tian, 下丹田). The second is in the area of the lower sternum, and is called the "Middle Dan Tian" (Zhong Dan Tian, 中丹田). The third is the lower center of forehead (or the third eye), connected to the brain and is called the "Upper Dan Tian" (Shang Dan Tian, 上丹田).

The Lower Dan Tian is considered to be the residence of the Water Qi, or the Qi which is generated from the Original Essence (Yuan Jing, 元精). Therefore, Qi stored here is called Original Qi (Yuan Qi, 元氣). According to Chinese medicine, in this same area there is a cavity called "Qihai"(Co-6)(氣海), which means "Qi ocean." This is consistent with the conclusions drawn by Qigong practitioners, who also call this area the "Lower Dan Tian" (lower elixir field). Both groups agree that this area is able to produce Qi or elixir like a field, and that here the Qi is abundant like an ocean.

In Qigong practice, it is commonly known that in order to build up the Qi to a higher level in the Lower Dan Tian, you must move your abdominal area (i.e., Lower Dan Tian) up and down through abdominal breathing. This kind of up and down abdominal breathing exercise is called "Qi Huo" (起火) and means "start the fire." It

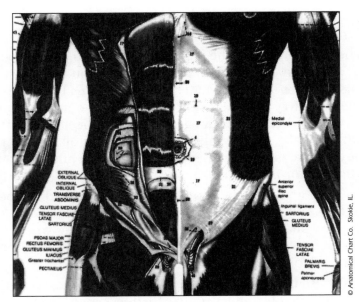

Figure 1-3. Anatomic Structure of the Abdominal Area

is also called "back to childhood breathing" (Fan Tong Hu Xi, 返童呼吸). Normally, after you have exercised the Lower Dan Tian for about ten minutes, you will have a feeling of warmth in the lower abdomen, which implies the accumulation of Qi or energy.

Theoretically and scientifically, what is happening when the abdominal area is moved up and down? If you look at the structure of the abdominal area, you will see that there are about six layers of muscle and fasciae sandwiching each other in this area (Figure 1-3). In fact, what you actually see is the sandwich of muscles and fat accumulated in the fasciae layers. When you move your abdomen up and down, you are actually using your mind to move the muscles, not the fat. Whenever there is a muscular contraction and relaxation, the fat slowly turns into bioelectricity. When this bioelectricity encounters resistance from the fasciae layers, it turns into heat. From this, you can see how simple the theory might be for the generation of Qi. Another thing you should know is that, according to our understanding today, fat and fasciae are poor electrical conductors, while the muscles are relatively good electrical conductors.[3, 4, & 5] When these good and poor electrical materials are sandwiched together, they act like a battery. This is why, through up and down abdominal movements, the energy can be stored temporarily and generate warmth.

However, through nearly two thousand years of experience, Daoists have said that the front abdominal area is not the real Dan Tian, but is in fact a "False Dan Tian" (Jia Dan Tian, 假丹田). Their argument is that, although this Lower Dan Tian is able to generate Qi and build it up to a higher level, it does not store it for a long time. This is because the Lower Dan Tian is located on the path of the Conception Vessel (please refer to the next chapter about vessels), so that whenever Qi is built up to a higher energetic state, it will circulate in the Conception and Governing Vessels.

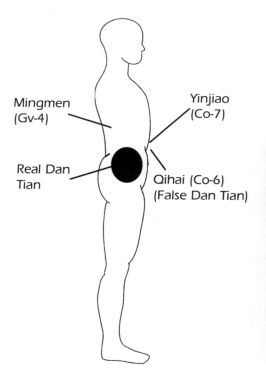

Mingmen
(Gv-4)

Yinjiao
(Co-7)

Real Dan
Tian

Qihai (Co-6)
(False Dan Tian)

**Figure 1-4. The Real Dan Tian
and the False Dan Tian**

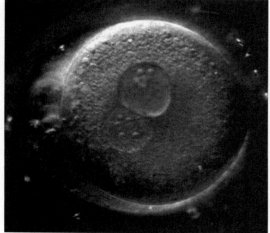

Figure 1-5. Original First Human Cell

According to Chinese medicine, these two vessels regulate and govern the Qi conditions in the body's twelve primary Qi channels. Therefore, when there is any extra Qi in these two vessels, it will eventually redistribute to the entire body through the twelve channels. This Lower Dan Tian therefore cannot be a battery as we understand the term. A real battery should be able to store the Qi. Where then, is the "Real Dan Tian" (Zhen Dan Tian, 眞丹田)?

Daoists teach that the Real Dan Tian is at the center of the abdominal area, at the physical center of the gravity located in the large and small intestines (Figure 1-4). Now, let us analyze this from two different points of view.

First, let us take a look of how a life is started. It begins with a sperm from the father entering an egg from the mother, thus forming the original human cell (Figure 1-5).[6] This cell next divides into two cells, then four cells, etc. When this group of cells adheres to the internal wall of the uterus, the umbilical cord starts to develop. Nutrition and energy for further cell multiplication is absorbed through the umbilical cord from the mother's body. The baby keeps growing until matured. During this nourishing and growing process, the baby's abdomen is moving up and down, acting like a pump drawing in nutrition and energy into his or her body. Later, immediately after the birth, air and nutrition are taken in from the nose and mouth through the mouth's sucking action and the lungs' breathing. As the child grows, it slowly forgets the natural movements of the abdomen. This is why the abdomen's up and down movement is called "back to the childhood breathing."

Think carefully: if your first human cell is still alive, where is this cell? Naturally, this cell has already died a long time ago. It is understood that approximately one trillion (10^{12}) cells die in the human body each day[7]. However, if we assume that this first cell is still alive, then it should be located at our physical center, that is, our center of gravity. If we think carefully, we can see that it is from this center that the cells could multiply evenly outward until the body is completely constructed. In order to maintain this even multiplication physically, the energy or Qi must be centered at this point and radiate outward. When we are in an embryonic state, this is the gravity center and also the Qi center. As we grow after birth, this center remains.

The above argument adheres solely to the traditional point of view of the physical development of our body. Next, let us analyze this center from another point of view.

If we look at the physical center of gravity, we can see that the entire area is occupied by the Large and Small intestines (Figure 1-6). We know that there are three kinds of muscles existing in our body, and can examine them in ascending order of our ability to control them. The first kind is the heart muscle, in which the electrical conductivity among muscular groups is the highest. The heart beats all the time, regardless of our attention, and through practice and discipline, we are able only to regulate its beating, not start and stop it. If we supply electricity to even a small piece of this muscle, it will pump like the heart. The second category of muscles are those which contract automatically but slowly, such as the muscles in the Large and Small intestines, and their electrical conductivity is lower than the first type. The third kind of muscles are those muscles which are directly controlled by our conscious mind. The electric conductivity of these muscles is the lowest of the three groups.

If you look at the structure of the Large and Small Intestines, the first thing you notice is that the total length of your Large and Small Intestines is approximately six times your body's height (Figure 1-7). With such long electrically conductive tissues sandwiched between all of the mesentery, water, and outer casings (which it is reasonable to believe are poor electrical conductive tissues), it acts like a huge battery in our body (Figure 1-8).[8] From this, you can see that it makes sense both logically and scientifically that the center of gravity, rather than the false Dan Tian, is the real battery in our body.

Next, let us examine the structure of the Middle Dan Tian area. The Middle Dan Tian is located next to the diaphragm (Figure 1-9). We know that the diaphragm is a membranous muscular partition separating the abdominal and the thoracic cavities. It functions in respiration and is a good electrically conductive material. On the top and the bottom of the diaphragm there is the fasciae, which isolates the internal organs from the diaphragm. We see now again a good electrical conductor isolated by a poor electrical conductor. That means that it is capable of storing electricity or Qi. Since this place is between the lungs and the stomach, and they absorb the Post-Birth essence (air and food) and convert it into energy, the Qi accumulated in the Middle Dan Tian is classified as Fire Qi. The reason for this name is that the Qi converted from the contaminated air and the food can affect Qi status and make it Yang.

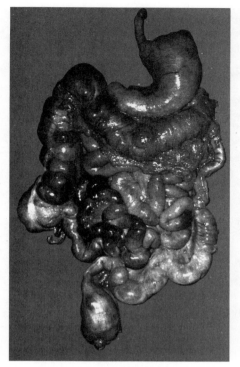

Figure 1-6. Anatomic Structure
of the Real Dan Tian

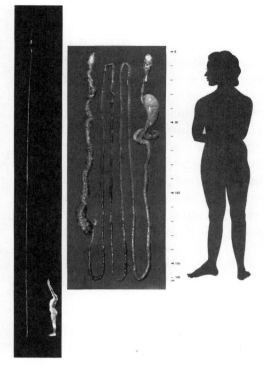

Figure 1-7. The Large and Small Intestines
are About Six Times Your Height

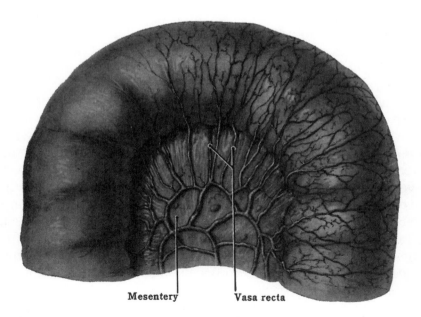

Mesentery   Vasa recta

Figure 1-8. Low Electrically Conductive Materials Such as Mesentery, Outer Casing, and Water
in and Around the Intestines Makes the Entire Area Act Like a Battery

(James E. Anderson, M.D., Grant's Atlas of Anatomy, 7th ed., © Williams & Wilkins)

Naturally, this Fire Qi can also agitate your emotional mind.

Finally, let us analyze the brain, which is considered the Upper Dan Tian. We already know that the brain and the spinal cord are considered to be the central nervous system, in which the electrical conductivity is highest in our body. If we examine the brain's structure, we can see that it is segregated by the arachnoid mater (i.e., a delicate membrane of the spinal cord and brain, lying between the pia mater and dura mater) into separate portions (Figure 1-10). It is reasonable to assume that these materials are low electrically conductive tissues. Again, it is another giant battery which consumes Qi in great amounts. However, since the brain does not produce Qi or bioelectricity, its function as a Dan Tian cannot be considered to be the same as the Lower Dan Tian.

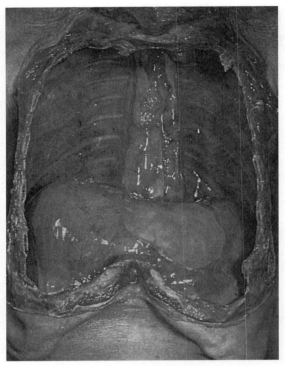

Figure 1-9. The Middle Dan Tian is Connected to the Diaphragm

From the above discussion, you may have gained a better idea of how we can link ancient experience together with modern scientific understanding. Recently, scientists have even discovered that we have two "brains" coexisting in our body. One is the head, as we have known for quite some time. The other is actually in the gut. These scientists have confirmed that the upper brain is able to think and store memory. However, the lower brain is believed capable of storing memory only. These two brains are connected and communicate with each other through the spinal cord (i.e., Thrusting Vessel), a very highly electrically conductive nerve fiber. Therefore, while physically there are two brains, in function, they act as one unit. The upper brain thinks and generates EMF, and the lower brain stores charges and supplies electricity through the spinal cord.[9]

This is very consistent with the Chinese discoveries discussed earlier. As mentioned previously, according to Chinese Qigong, the upper brain is our Upper Dan Tian, where the spirit resides and the mind functions, while the Lower Dan Tian in the gut (i.e., stomach, large and small intestines) is the place which stores and supplies Qi. From this, you can clearly see that both Chinese empirical experience and modern science agree that the more you can concentrate, the higher your EMF will be. This will lead to more electricity being led from the Lower Dan Tian through the spinal cord (i.e., Thrusting Vessel) to anywhere in your physical body for action.

In order to make the scientific concept of Qigong even more clear, let us look at Qigong from another scientific point of view, this time chemical.

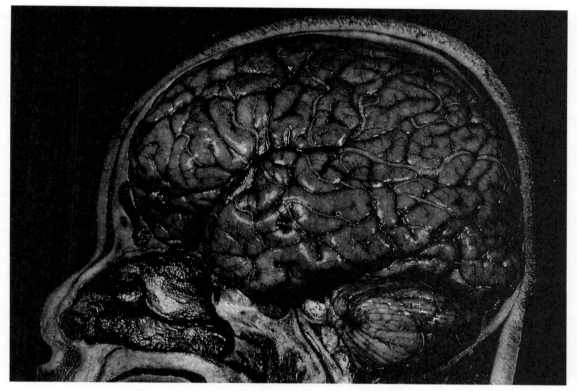

Figure 1-10. The Upper Dan Tian—The Human Brain

If we examine how we breath, we can see that we inhale to take in oxygen, and we exhale to expel carbon dioxide (Figure 1-11). From this, we can see that every minute we expel a great deal of carbon from our body through exhalation. Carbon is a material in a physical form which can be seen. The question is, where is the carbon coming from in our body? Through breathing, how much carbon is actually processed out?

The first source of carbon is from the food (glucose) we eat. When this food is converted into energy through chemical reaction during our daily activities, carbon dioxide is produced.[10]

$$\text{glucose} + 6O_2 \rightarrow 6\ CO_2 + 6H_2O$$
$$\Delta G^{\circ\prime} = -686 \text{ kcal}$$

The second source of this carbon is from the dead cells in our body. We already know that the majority of our body is constructed from the elements carbon (C), hydrogen (H_2), oxygen (O_2), and nitrogen (N_2), while other elements such as Calcium (Ca), Phosphorus (P), Chloride (Cl), Sulfur (S), Potassium (K), Sodium (Na), Magnesium (Mg), Iodine (I), and Iron (Fe) comprise much less of our body weight. This means that the cells in our body contain a great amount of carbon.

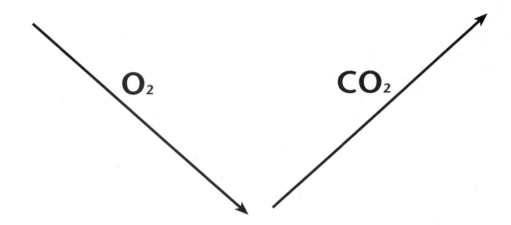

Figure 1-11. We Inhale to Absorb Oxygen and Exhale to Expel Carbon Dioxide

In addition, consider that every cell in our body has a lifetime. As many as a trillion (10^{12}) cells die in our body every twenty four hours.[7] For example, we know that the life span of a skin cell is twenty eight days. Naturally, every living cell such as those of the bone, marrow, liver, etc. have their own individual lifetime. We rely on our respiration to bring the carbon (i.e., dead cells) out, and to supply living cells with new oxygen through inhalation, and new carbon sources, water, and other minerals from eating. All this aids in the formation of new cells and the continuation of life.

From the foregoing, we can conclude that the cell replacement process is ongoing at all times in our life. Health during our lifetime depends on how smoothly and how quickly this replacement process is carried out. If there are more new healthy cells to replace the old cells, you live and grow. If the cells replaced are as healthy as the original cells, you remain young. However, if there are fewer cells produced, or if the new cells are not as healthy as the original cells, then you age. Now, let us analyze Qigong from the point of view of cell replacement.

In order to produce a good, healthy cell, first you must consider the materials which are needed. From the structure of a cell, we know that we will need hydrogen, oxygen, carbon, and other minerals which we can absorb either from air or food. Therefore, air quality, water purity, and the choice of foods become critical factors for your health and longevity. Naturally, this has also been a big component of Qigong study.

However, we know that air and water quality today has been contaminated by pollution. This is especially bad in big cities and industrial areas. The quality of the food we eat depends on their source and processing methods. Naturally, it is not easy to find the same pristine environments as in ancient times. However, we must learn how to fit into our new environment and choose the way of our life wisely.

Since carbon comprises such a major part of our body, how to absorb good quality carbon is an important issue in modern health. You may obtain carbon from animal products or from plants. Generally speaking, the carbon taken from plants is more pure and clean than that taken from animals.

According to past experience and analysis, red meat is generally more contaminated than white meat, and is able to disturb and stimulate your emotional mind and confuse your thinking. Another source from which animal products can be obtained is fish. Again, some fish are good and others may be bad. For example, shrimp is high in cholesterol, which may increase your risk of high blood pressure.

Due to the impurities contained in most animal products, since ancient times Qigong practitioners learned how to absorb protein from plants, especially from peas or beans. Soy bean is one of the best of these sources; it is both inexpensive and easy to grow. However, if you are not a vegetarian originally, then it can be difficult for your body to produce the enzymes to digest an all-vegetable diet immediately. Humans evolved as omnivores, and the craving for meat can be strong. Even today, we all still have canine teeth, which are designed for the simple purpose of tearing flesh from bone. Therefore, the natural enzymes existing in our body are more tailored to digesting meat. In an experiment, if we place a piece of meat and some corn in human digestive enzymes, we will see that the meat will be dissolved in a matter of minutes, while the corn will take many hours. This means it is generally easier for a human to absorb meat rather than plants as a protein source.

However, the above discussion does not mean we cannot absolutely absorb plant protein efficiently. The key is that if it is present to begin with, the **enzyme production can be increased within your body**, but it will take time. For example, if you cannot drink milk due to insufficient lactate in your stomach, you may start by drinking a little bit of milk every day, and slowly increase it as days pass by. You will realize that you can absorb milk six months later. This means that if you wish to become a vegetarian, you must reduce the intake of meat products slowly and allow your body to adjust to it; otherwise you may experience protein deficiency.

Other than a protein source, you must also consider minerals. Although they do not comprise a large proportion of our body, their importance in some ways is more significant than carbon. We know that calcium is an important element for bones, and iron is crucial for blood cells, etc. Therefore, when we eat we must consume a variety of foods instead of just a few. How to absorb nutrition from food has been an important part of Chinese Qigong study.

In order to produce healthy cells, other than the concerns of the material side, you must also consider energy. You should understand that when a person ages quickly, often it is not because he or she is malnourished, but instead is due to the weakening of their Qi storage and circulation. Without an abundant supply of Qi (bioelectricity), Qi circulation will not be regulated efficiently, and therefore your life force will weaken and the physical body will degenerate. In order to have abundant Qi storage, you must learn Qigong in order to build up the Qi in your eight vessels, and also to help you understand how to lead the Qi circulating in your body. This kind of Qigong training includes Wai Dan (external elixir, 外丹) and Nei Dan (internal elixir, 內丹) practice, which we will discuss in the next section.

Other than the concern for materials needed, and the Qi required for cell production and replacement, the next thing you should ask yourself is how this replacement process is carried out. Then, you will see that the entire replacement process depends on the blood cells. From Western medicine, we know that a blood cell is the carrier of water, oxygen, and nutrients to everywhere in the body through the blood circulatory network. From arteries and capillaries, the components for new cells are brought to every tiny place in the body. The old cells then absorb everything required from the blood stream and divide to produce new cells. The dead cells are brought back through veins to the lungs. Through respiration, the dead cell materials are expelled from the body as carbon dioxide.

However, there is one thing missing from the last process. This is the Qi or bio-electricity which is required for the biochemical process of cell division. It has been proven that every blood cell is actually like a dipole or a small battery, which is able to store bioelectricity and also to release it.[3] This means that each blood cell is actually a carrier of Qi. This is also understood in Chinese medicine. In Chinese medicine, the blood and the Qi are always together. Where there is blood, there is Qi, and where there is Qi, the blood will also be there. Therefore, the term "Qi-Xue" (i.e., Qi-blood)(氣血) is often used in Chinese medicine.

If you understand the above discussion, and if we take a look at our blood circulatory system, we can see that the arteries are located deeply underneath the muscles, while the veins are situated near the skin's surface. The color of the blood is red in the arteries because of the presence of oxygen, and its color is blue in the veins both because of the absence of this oxygen and the presence of carbon dioxide. This implies that cell replacement actually happens from inside of the body, moving outward. This can also offer us a hint that, if we tense more, the blood circulation will be more stagnant, and cell replacement will be slower. We can also conclude that most cell replacement occurs in the night when we are at our most relaxed state, during sleep. This can further lead one to conclude the importance of sleeping.

If we already know that blood cells are the carriers of everything which is required for cell replacement, then we must also consider the health of our blood cells. If you have good health and a sufficient quantity of blood cells, then the nutrition and Qi can be carried to every part of the body efficiently. You will be healthy. However, if you do not have sufficient blood cells, or if the quality of the cells is poor, then the entire cell replacement process will be stagnant. Naturally, you will degenerate swiftly.

According to modern medical science, blood cells also have a life span. When the old ones die, new ones must be produced from the bone marrow. Bone marrow is the major blood factory. From medical reports, we know that normally, after a person reaches thirty, the marrow near the ends of the bone cavity turns yellow. This indicates that fat has accumulated there. It also means that red blood cells are no longer being produced in the yellowed area (Figure 1-12).[11] Chinese Qigong practitioners believe that the degeneration of the bone marrow is due to insufficient Qi supply. Therefore, Bone Marrow Washing Qigong was developed. From experience, through marrow washing Qigong practice, health can be improved and life can be extended significantly. If you are interested in this subject, please read *Muscle/Tendon Changing and Marrow/Brain Washing Chi Kung*, from YMAA Publication Center.

In addition to the above, the next thing which is highly important in human life is hormone production within your body. We already know from today's medical science that hormones act as a catalyst in the body. When the hormone levels are high, we are more energized and cell replacement can happen faster and more smoothly. When hormone production is slow and its level is low, then the cell replacement will be slow and we will age quickly. It is only in the last few years that scientists have discovered that by increasing the hormone levels in the body, we may be able to extend our life significantly.[12]

Maintenance of hormone production in a healthy manner has also been a major concern in Chinese Qigong practice. According to Chinese medicine, glands which produce hormones were recognized since ancient times. Hormones were not understood. However, throughout a thousand years of practice and experience, it was understood that the essence of life is stored in the kidneys. Today, we know that this essence is actually the hormones produced from the adrenal glands

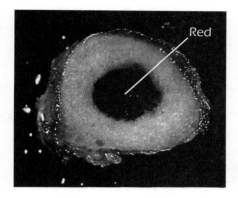

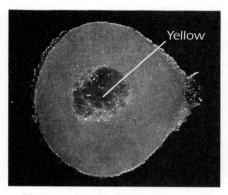

Figure 1-12. Structure of a Long Bone. Red Bone Marrow and Yellow Bone Marrow

on the top of the kidneys. The Chinese also believed that through stimulation of the testicles and ovaries, the life force could be increased. In addition, from still meditation practice, they learned how to lead the Qi to the brain and raise up the "spirit of vitality." It has also been found that through practice, bioelectricity can be led to the pituitary gland to stimulate growth hormone production. All of these practices are believed to be effective paths to longevity.

From medical science, we know that our hormone levels are significantly reduced when the last pieces of our bones are completed, between ages 29 to 30. Theoretically, when our body has completed constructing itself, it somehow triggers the reduction of our hormone levels. From this, you can see that maintaining the hormone levels in our body may be a key to longevity.

Finally, in order to prevent ourselves from getting sick, we must also consider our immune system. According to Chinese medicine and Qigong, when Qi storage is abundant, you get sick less. If we take a careful look, we can realize that every white blood cell is just like a fighting soldier. If we do not have enough Qi to supply it, its fighting capability will be low. It is just like a soldier who needs food to maintain his strength. When the Qi is strong, the immune system is strong. Therefore, the skin breathing technique has been developed, which teaches a practitioner to lead the Qi to the surface of the skin to strengthen the "Guardian Qi" (Wei Qi, 衛氣) or an energetic component of the immune system near the skin surface.

From the foregoing, hopefully I have offered you a challenge for profound thought and understanding. Although most of these conclusions are drawn from my personal research, further study and verification is still needed. I deeply believe that if we can all open our minds and share our opinions together, we will be able to make our lives more healthy and meaningful.

1-3. The History of Qigong

The history of Chinese Qigong can be roughly divided into four periods. We know little about the first period, which is considered to have started when the *Yi Jing (Book of Changes)* was introduced sometime before 1122 B.C., and to have extended until the Han dynasty (206 B.C., 漢) when Buddhism and its meditation methods were imported from India. This infusion brought Qigong practice and meditation into the second period, the religious Qigong era. This period lasted until the Liang dynasty (502-557 A.D., 梁), when it was discovered that Qigong could be used for martial purposes. This was the beginning of the third period, that of martial Qigong. Many different martial Qigong styles were created based on the theories and principles of Buddhist and Daoist Qigong. This period lasted until the overthrow of the Qing (清) dynasty in 1911; from that point Chinese Qigong training was mixed with Qigong practices from India, Japan, and many other countries.

Before the Han Dynasty (Before 206 B.C., 漢前)

The *Yi Jing* (*Book of Changes*; 1122 B.C.) was probably the first Chinese book related to Qi. It introduced the concept of the three natural energies or powers (San Cai, 三才): Tian (Heaven, 天), Di (Earth, 地), and Ren (Man, 人). Studying the relationship of these three natural powers was the first step in the development of Qigong.

From 1766-1154 B.C. (the Shang dynasty, 商), the Chinese capital was located in today's An Yang in Henan province (河南，安陽). An archaeological dig there, at a late Shang dynasty burial ground called Yin Xu (殷墟), discovered more than 160,000 pieces of turtle shell and animal bone which were covered with written characters. This writing, called *Jia Gu Wen* (Oracle-Bone Scripture, 甲骨文), is the earliest evidence of the Chinese use of the written word. Most of the information recorded was of a religious nature. Together with these oracle-bone scriptures were discovered the so called Bian Shi (stone probes, 砭石)(Figure 1-13). The name Bian Shi was recorded in the *Nei Jing (Inner Classic,* 內經), which mentioned that during the reign of the Yellow emperor (2690-2590 B.C., 黃帝) Bian Shi were already being used to adjust people's Qi circulation.

During the Zhou dynasty (1122-934 B.C.), Lao Zi (Li Er) mentioned certain breathing techniques in his classic *Dao De Jing* (or *Tao Te Ching,* 道德經) (*Classic on the*

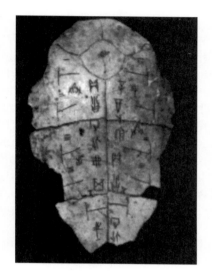
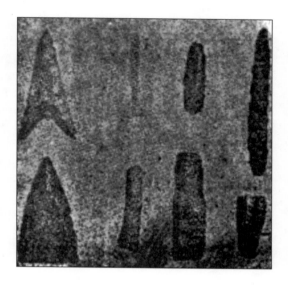

Figure 1-13. Jia Gu Wen (Oracle-Bone Scripture) and Bian Shi (Stone Probes)

Virtue of the Dao). He stressed that the way to obtain health was to "concentrate on Qi and achieve softness" (Zhuan Qi Zhi Rou, 專氣致柔). Later, *Shi Ji* (*Historical Record*, 史紀) in the Spring and Autumn and Warring States Periods (770-221 B.C., 春秋戰國) also described more complete methods of breath training. About 300 B.C. the Daoist philosopher Zhuang Zi (莊子) described the relationship between health and the breath in his book *Nan Hua Jing* (南華經). It states: "The real person's (i.e., immortal's) breathing reaches down to their heels. The normal person's breathing is in the throat."[13] This suggests that a breathing method for Qi circulation was already being used by some Daoists at that time.

During the Qin and Han dynasties (221 B.C.-220 A.D., 秦，漢) there are several medical references to Qigong in the literature, such as the *Nan Jing* (*Classic on Disorders*, 難經) by the famous physician Bian Que (扁鵲), which describes using the breathing to increase Qi circulation. *Jin Kui Yao Lue* (*Prescriptions from the Golden Chamber,* 金匱要略) by Zhang, Zhong-Jing (張仲景) discusses the use of breathing and acupuncture to maintain good Qi flow. *Zhou Yi Can Tong Qi* (*A Comparative Study of the Zhou (dynasty) Book of Changes,* 周易參同契) by Wei, Bo-Yang (魏伯陽) explains the relationship of human beings to nature's forces and Qi. It can be seen from this list that up to this time, almost all of the Qigong publications were written by scholars such as Lao Zi (老子) and Zhuang Zi (莊子), or physicians such as Bian Que and Wei, Bo-Yang.

From the Han Dynasty to the Beginning of the Liang Dynasty
(206 B.C.-502 A.D.)(漢 - 梁)

Because many Han emperors were intelligent and wise, the Han dynasty was a glorious and peaceful period. It was during the Eastern Han dynasty (c. 58 A.D., 東漢) that Buddhism was imported to China from India. The Han emperor became a sincere Buddhist; Buddhism soon spread and became very popular. Many Buddhist meditation and Qigong practices, which had been practiced in India for thousands of years, were absorbed into the Chinese culture. The Buddhist temples taught many Qigong practices, especially the still meditation of Chan (Zen)(禪，忍), which marked a new era of Chinese Qigong. Much of the deeper Qigong theory and practices which had been developed in India were brought to China. Unfortunately, since the training was directed at attaining Buddhahood, the training practices and theory were recorded in the Buddhist bibles and kept secret. For hundreds of years the religious Qigong training was never taught to laymen. Only in this century has it been available to the general populace.

Not long after Buddhism had been imported into China, a Daoist by the name of Zhang, Dao-Ling (張道陵) combined the traditional Daoist principles with Buddhism and created a religion called Dao Jiao (道教). Many of the meditation methods were a combination of the principles and training methods of both sources.

Since Tibet had developed its own branch of Buddhism with its own training system and methods of attaining Buddhahood, Tibetan Buddhists were also invited to China to preach. In time, their practices were also absorbed.

It was in this period that the traditional Chinese Qigong practitioners finally had a chance to compare their arts with the religious Qigong practices imported mainly from India. While the scholarly and medical Qigong had been concerned with maintaining and improving health, the newly imported religious Qigong was concerned with far more. Contemporary documents and Qigong styles show clearly that the religious practitioners trained their Qi to a much deeper level, working with many internal functions of the body, and strove to obtain control of their bodies, minds, and spirits with the goal of escaping from the cycle of reincarnation.

While the Qigong practices and meditations were being passed down secretly within the monasteries, traditional scholars and physicians continued their Qigong research. During the Jin dynasty (晉) in the 3rd century A.D., a famous physician named Hua Tuo (華陀) used acupuncture for anesthesia in surgery. The Daoist Jun Qian (君倩) used the movements of animals to create the Wu Qin Xi (Five Animal Sports, 五禽戲), which taught people how to increase their Qi circulation through specific movements (some say that the Wu Qin Xi was created by Hua Tuo). Also, in this period a physician named Ge Hong (葛洪) mentioned using the mind to lead and increase Qi in his book *Bao Pu Zi* (抱朴子). Sometime in the period of 420 to 581 A.D. Tao, Hong-Jing (陶弘景) compiled the *Yang Shen Yan Ming Lu* (*Records of Nourishing the Body and Extending Life*, 養身延命錄), which showed many Qigong techniques.

From the Liang Dynasty to the End of the Qing Dynasty (502-1911 A.D.)(梁 - 清)

During the Liang dynasty (502-557 A.D., 梁) the emperor invited a Buddhist monk named Da Mo (達磨), who was once an Indian prince, to preach Buddhism in China. The emperor decided he did not like Da Mo's Buddhist theory, so the monk withdrew to the Shaolin Temple (少林寺). When Da Mo arrived, he saw that the priests were weak and sickly, so he shut himself away to ponder the problem. He emerged after nine years of seclusion and wrote two classics: *Yi Jin Jing (Muscle/Tendon Changing Classic*, 易筋經) and *Xi Sui Jing (Marrow/Brain Washing Classic*, 洗髓經). The *Muscle/Tendon Changing Classic* taught the priests how to gain health and change their physical bodies from weak to strong. The *Marrow/Brain Washing Classic* taught the priests how to use Qi to clean the bone marrow and strengthen the blood and immune system, as well as how to energize the brain and attain enlightenment. Because the *Marrow/Brain Washing Classic* was harder to understand and practice, the training methods were passed down secretly to only a very few disciples in each generation.

After the priests practiced the Muscle/Tendon Changing exercises, they found that not only did they improve their health, but they also greatly increased their strength. When this training was integrated into the martial arts forms, it increased the effectiveness of their techniques. In addition to this martial Qigong training, the Shaolin priests also created five animal styles of Gongfu which imitated the way different animals fight. The animals imitated were the tiger, leopard, dragon, snake, and crane.

Outside of the monastery, the development of Qigong continued during the Sui and Tang dynasties (581-907 A.D., 隋，唐). Chao, Yuan-Fang (巢元方) compiled the *Zhu Bing Yuan Hou Lun (Thesis on the Origins and Symptoms of Various Diseases*, 諸病源候論), which is a veritable encyclopedia of Qigong methods, listing 260 different ways of increasing the Qi flow. The *Qian Jin Fang (Thousand Gold Prescriptions*, 千金方) by Sun, Si-Mao (孫思邈) described the method of leading Qi, and also described the use of the Six Sounds. The Buddhists and Daoists had already been using the Six Sounds to regulate Qi in the internal organs for some time. Sun Si-Mao also introduced a massage system called Lao Zi's 49 Massage Techniques. *Wai Tai Mi Yao (The Extra Important Secret*, 外台祕要) by Wang Tao (王燾) discussed the use of breathing and herbal therapies for disorders of Qi circulation.

During the Song, Jin, and Yuan dynasties (960-1368 A.D., 宋，金，元), *Yang Shen Jue (Life Nourishing Secrets*, 養生訣) by Zhang, An-Dao (張安道) discussed several Qigong practices. *Ru Men Shi Shi (The Confucian Point of View*, 儒門視事) by Zhang, Zi-He (張子和) describes the use of Qigong to cure external injuries such as cuts and sprains. *Lan Shi Mi Cang (Secret Library of the Orchid Room*, 蘭室祕藏) by Li Guo (李果) describes using Qigong and herbal remedies for internal disorders. *Ge Zhi Yu Lun (A Further Thesis of Complete Study*, 格致餘論) by Zhu, Dan-Xi (朱丹溪) provided a theoretical explanation for the use of Qigong in curing disease.

During the Song dynasty (960-1279 A.D., 宋), Chang, San-Feng (張三豐) is believed to have created Taijiquan (or Tai Chi Chuan, 太極拳). Taiji followed a different approach in its use of Qigong than did Shaolin. While Shaolin emphasized Wai Dan (External Elixir, 外丹) Qigong exercises, Taiji emphasized Nei Dan (Internal Elixir, 内丹) Qigong training.

In 1026 A.D. the famous brass man of acupuncture was designed and built by Dr. Wang, Wei-Yi (王唯一). Before that time, the many publications which discussed acupuncture theory, principles, and treatment techniques disagreed with each other, and left many points unclear. When Dr. Wang built his brass man, he also wrote a book called *Tong Ren Yu Xue Zhen Jiu Tu* (*Illustration of the Brass Man Acupuncture and Moxibustion*, 銅人俞穴鍼灸圖). He explained the relationship of the 12 organs and the 12 Qi channels, clarified many of the points of confusion, and, for the first time, systematically organized acupuncture theory and principles.

In 1034 A.D. Dr. Wang used acupuncture to cure the emperor Ren Zong (仁宗). With the support of the emperor, acupuncture flourished. In order to encourage acupuncture medical research, the emperor built a temple to Bian Que, who wrote the *Nan Jing*, and worshipped him as the ancestor of acupuncture. Acupuncture technology developed so much that even the Jin race in the distant North requested the brass man and other acupuncture technology as a condition for peace. Between 1102 to 1106 A.D. Dr. Wang dissected the bodies of prisoners and added more information to the *Nan Jing*. His work contributed greatly to the advancement of Qigong and Chinese medicine by giving a clear and systematic idea of the circulation of Qi in the human body.

Later, in the Southern Song dynasty (1127-1279 A.D., 南宋), Marshal Yue Fei (岳飛) was credited with creating several internal Qigong exercises and martial arts. It is said that he created Ba Duan Jin (The Eight Pieces of Brocade, 八段錦) to improve the health of his soldiers. He is also known as the creator of the internal martial style Xingyi (形意). Eagle style martial artists also claim that Yue Fei was the creator of their style.

From then until the end of the Qing dynasty (1911 A.D., 清), many other Qigong styles were founded. The well known ones include Hu Bu Gong (Tiger Step Gong, 虎步功), Shi Er Zhuang (Twelve Postures, 十二庄) and Jiao Hua Gong (Beggar Gong, 叫化功). Also in this period, many documents related to Qigong were published, such as *Bao Shen Mi Yao* (*The Secret Important Document of Body Protection*, 保身祕要) by Cao, Yuan-Bai (曹元白), which described moving and stationary Qigong practices; and *Yang Shen Fu Yu* (*Brief Introduction to Nourishing the Body*, 養生膚語) by Chen, Ji-Ru (陳繼儒), about the three treasures: Jing (essence, 精), Qi (internal energy, 氣), and Shen (spirit, 神). Also, *Yi Fan Ji Jie* (*The Total Introduction to Medical Prescriptions*, 醫方集介) by Wang, Fan-An (汪汎庵) reviewed and summarized the previously published materials; and *Nei Gong Tu Shuo* (*Illustrated Explanation of Nei Gong*, 内功圖説) by Wang, Zu-Yuan (王祖源) presented the Twelve Pieces of Brocade and explained the idea of combining both moving and stationary Qigong.

In the late Ming dynasty (around 1640 A.D., 明), a martial Qigong style, Huo Long Gong (Fire Dragon Gong, 火龍功), was created by the Taiyang martial stylists (太陽宗). The well known internal martial art style Baguazhang (Eight Trigrams Palm,

八卦掌) is believed to have been created by Dong, Hai-Chuan (董海川) late in the Qing dynasty (1644-1911 A.D., 清). This style is now gaining in popularity throughout the world.

During the Qing dynasty, Tibetan meditation and martial techniques became widespread in China for the first time. This was due to the encouragement and interest of the Manchurian Emperors in the royal palace, as well as others of high rank in society.

From the End of Qing Dynasty to the Present (清後)

Before 1911 A.D., Chinese society was still very conservative and old-fashioned. Even though China had been expanding its contact with the outside world for the previous hundred years, the outside world had little influence beyond the coastal regions. With the overthrow of the Qing dynasty in 1911 and the founding of the Chinese Republic, the nation began changing as never before. Since this time Qigong practice has entered a new era. Because of the ease of communication in the modern world, Western culture now has great influence on the Orient. Many Chinese have opened their minds and changed their traditional ideas, especially in Taiwan and Hong Kong. Various Qigong styles are now being taught openly, and many formerly secret documents have been published. Modern methods of communication have opened up Qigong to a much wider audience than ever before, and people now have the opportunity to study and understand many different styles. In addition, people are now able to compare Chinese Qigong to similar arts from other countries such as India, Japan, Korea, and the Middle East.

I believe that in the near future Qigong will be considered the most exciting and challenging field of research. It is an ancient science just waiting to be investigated with the help of the new technologies now being developed at an almost explosive rate. Anything we can do to speed up this research will greatly help humanity to understand and improve itself.

1-4. Categories of Qigong

Often, people ask me the same question: Is jogging, weight lifting, or dancing a kind of Qigong practice? To answer this question, let us trace back Qigong history to before the Chinese Qin and Han dynastic periods (255 B.C.-223 A.D., 秦，漢). Then you can see that the origins of many Qigong practices were actually in dancing. Through dancing, the physical body was exercised and the health of the physical body was maintained. Also, through dancing and matching movements with music, the mind was regulated into a harmonious state. From this harmonious mind, the spirit can be raised to a more energized state, or can be calmed down to a peaceful level. This Qigong dancing later passed to Japan during the Chinese Han Dynasty, and became a very elegant, slow, and high style of dancing in the Japanese royal court. This Taijiquan-like dancing is still practiced in Japan today.

Phyisical
(Yang)

Mind
(Yin)

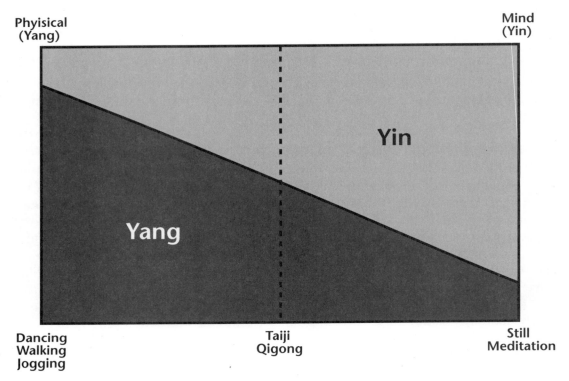

Dancing
Walking
Jogging

Taiji
Qigong

Still
Meditation

Figure 1-14. The Range of Defined Qigong

The ways of African or Native American dancing in which the body is bounced up and down is also known as a means of loosening up the joints and improving Qi circulation. Naturally, jogging, weight lifting, or even walking are a kind of Qigong practice. Therefore, we can say that **any activity which is able to regulate the Qi circulation** in the body is a Qigong practice.

Let us define it more clearly. In Figure 1-14, if the left vertical line represents the amount of usage of the physical body (Yang, 陽), and the right vertical line is the usage of the mind (Yin, 陰), then we can see that the more you practice toward the left, the more physical effort, and the less mind, is needed. This can be aerobic dancing, walking, or jogging in which the mind usage is relatively little compared to physical action. In this kind of Qigong practice, normally you do not need special training, and it is classified as layman Qigong. In the middle point, the mind and the physical activity are almost equally important. This kind of Qigong will be the slow Moving Qigong, in which the mind is used to lead the Qi in coordination with the movements. For example, Taiji Qigong, The Eight Pieces of Brocade, The Five Animal Sports, and many others are very typical Qigong exercises, especially in Chinese medical and martial arts societies.

However, when you reach a profound level of Qigong practice, the mind becomes more critical and important. When you reach this high level, you are dealing with your mind while you are sitting still. Most of this mental Qigong training was practiced by the scholars and religious Qigong practitioners. In this practice, you may have a little physical movement in the lower abdomen. However, the main focus of this Qigong practice is in the peaceful mind or spiritual enlightenment which originates from the cultivation of your mind. This kind of Qigong practice includes Sitting Chan (Ren) (坐禪，忍), Small Circulation Meditation (Xiao Zhou Tian, 小周天), Grand Circulation Meditation (Da Zhou Tian, 大周天), or Brain Washing Enlightenment Meditation (Xi Sui Gong, 洗髓功).

Theoretically speaking, in order to have good health, you will need to maintain your physical condition and also build up abundant Qi in your body. The best Qigong for health is actually located in the middle of our model, where you learn how to regulate your physical body and also your mind. From this Yin and Yang practice, your Qi can be circulated smoothly in the body.

Let us now review the traditional concepts of how Qigong was categorized. Generally speaking, all Qigong practices can be divided, according to their training theory and methods, into two general categories: Wai Dan (External Elixir, 外丹) and Nei Dan (Internal Elixir, 內丹). Understanding the differences between them will give you an overview of most Chinese Qigong practice.

External and Internal Elixirs

Wai Dan (External Elixir) 外丹. "Wai" means "external" or "outside," and "Dan" means "elixir." External here means the skin surface of the body or the limbs, as opposed to the torso or the center of the body, which includes all of the vital organs. Elixir is a hypothetical, life-prolonging substance for which Chinese Daoists have been searching for several millennia. They originally thought that the elixir was something physical which could be prepared from herbs or chemicals purified in a furnace. After thousands of years of study and experimentation, they found that the elixir is in the body. In other words, if you want to prolong your life, you must find the elixir in your body, and then learn to cultivate, protect, and nourish it. Actually, the elixir is what we have understood the inner energy or Qi circulating in the body to be.

There are many ways of producing elixir or Qi in the body. For example, in Wai Dan Qigong practice, you may exercise your limbs through dancing or even walking. As you exercise, the Qi builds up in your arms and legs. When the Qi potential in your limbs builds to a high enough level, the Qi will flow through the channels, clearing any obstructions and flowing into the center of the body to nourish the organs. This is the main reason that a person who works out, or has a physical job is, generally healthier than someone who sits around all day.

Naturally, you may simply massage your body to produce the Qi. Through massage, you may stimulate the cells of your body to a higher energized state and therefore the Qi concentration will be raised and the circulation enhanced. Then, after massage you relax, and the higher levels of Qi on the skin surface and muscles will flow into the center of the body and thereby improve the Qi circulatory conditions in your internal organs. This is the theoretical foundation of the Tui Na Qigong massage (pushing and grabbing massage, 推拿).

Through acupuncture, you may also bring the Qi level near the skin surface to a higher level and from this stimulation, the Qi condition of the internal organs can be regulated through Qi channels. Therefore, acupuncture can also be classified as Wai Dan Qigong practice. Naturally, the herbal treatments are a way of Wai Dan practice as well.

From this, we can briefly conclude that any possible stimulation or exercises which accumulate a high level of Qi on the surface of the body, and then flow inward toward the center of the body, can be classified as Wai Dan (external elixir)(Figure 1-15).

Nei Dan (Internal Elixir) 內丹 . "Nei" means "internal" and "Dan" again means "elixir." Thus, Nei Dan means to build the elixir internally. Here, internally means inside the torso, instead of on the limbs. Normally, the Qi is built on the Qi vessels instead of the primary Qi channels. Whereas in Wai Dan the Qi is built up in the limbs or skin surface and then moved into the body through primary Qi channels, Nei Dan exercises build up Qi in the torso and lead it out to the limbs (Figure 1-16).

Generally, speaking, Nei Dan theory is deeper than Wai Dan theory, and it is more difficult to understand and practice. Traditionally, most of the Nei Dan Qigong practices have been passed down more secretly than those of the Wai Dan. This is especially true of the highest levels of Nei Dan, such as Marrow/Brain Washing, which were passed down to only a few trusted disciples.

Schools of Qigong Practice

We can also classify Qigong into four major categories according to the purpose or final goal of the training: A. maintaining health; B. curing sickness; C. martial arts; D. enlightenment or Buddhahood. This is only a rough breakdown, however, since almost every style of Qigong serves more than one of the above purposes. For example, although martial Qigong focuses on increasing fighting effectiveness, it can also improve your health. Daoist Qigong aims for longevity and enlightenment, but to reach this goal you need to be in good health and know how to cure sickness. Because of this multi-purpose aspect of the categories, it will be simpler to discuss their backgrounds rather than the goals of their training. Knowing the history and basic principles of each category will help you to understand Qigong more clearly.

Scholar Qigong—for Maintaining Health. In China before the Han Dynasty, there were two major schools of scholarship. One of them was created by Confucius (551-479 B.C.)(孔子) during the Spring and Autumn period. Later, his philosophy was popularized and elaborated upon by Mencius (372-289 B.C.)(孟子) in the Warring States Period. The scholars who practice his philosophy are commonly called Confucians or Confucianists (Ru Jia, 儒家). The key words to their basic philosophy are **Loyalty** (Zhong, 忠), **Filial Piety** (Xiao, 孝), **Humanity** (Ren, 仁), **Kindness** (Ai, 愛), **Trust** (Xin, 信), **Justice** (Yi, 義), **Harmony** (He, 和), and **Peace** (Ping, 平). Humanity and human feelings are the main subjects of study. Ru Jia philosophy has become the center of much of Chinese culture.

The second major school of scholarship was called Dao Jia (Daoism)(道家) and was created by Lao Zi (老子) in the 6th century B.C. Lao Zi is considered to be

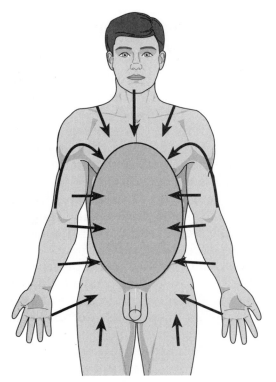

Figure 1-15. External Elixir (Wai Dan)

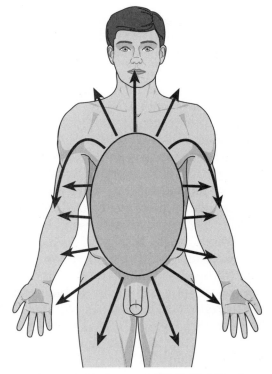

Figure 1-16. Internal Elixir (Nei Dan)

the author of a book called the *Dao De Jing* (*Classic on the Virtue of the Dao*)(道德經) which describes human morality. Later, in the Warring States Period, his follower Zhuang Zhou (莊周) wrote a book called *Zhuang Zi* (莊子) which led to the forming of another strong branch of Daoism. Before the Han Dynasty, Daoism was considered a branch of scholarship. However, in the Han Dynasty, traditional Daoism was combined with the Buddhism imported from India by Zhang, Dao-Ling (張道陵), and it began gradually to be treated as a religion. Therefore, the Daoism before the Han Dynasty should be considered scholarly Daoism rather than religious.

With regard to their contribution to Qigong, both schools emphasized maintaining health and preventing disease. They believed that many illnesses are caused by mental and emotional excesses. When a person's mind is not calm, balanced, and peaceful, the organs will not function normally. For example, depression can cause stomach ulcers and indigestion. Anger will cause the liver to malfunction. Sadness will cause stagnation and tightness in the lungs, and fear can disturb the normal functioning of the kidneys and bladder. They realized that if you want to avoid illness, you must learn to balance and relax your thoughts and emotions. This is called "regulating the mind" (Tiao Xin, 調心).

Therefore, the scholars emphasize gaining a peaceful mind through meditation. In their still meditation, the main part of the training is getting rid of thoughts so that the mind is clear and calm. When you become calm, the flow of thoughts and emotions slows down, and you feel mentally and emotionally neutral. This kind of meditation can be thought of as practicing emotional self-control. When you are in this "**no thought**" state, you become very relaxed, and can even relax deep down into your internal organs. When your body is this relaxed, your Qi will naturally flow smoothly and strongly. This kind of still meditation was very common in ancient China's scholarly society.

In order to reach the goal of a calm and peaceful mind, the scholars' training focused on regulating the mind, body, and breath. They believed that as long as these three things were regulated, the Qi flow would be smooth and sickness would not occur. This is why the Qi training of the scholars is called "Xiu Qi" (修氣), which means "cultivating Qi." "Xiu" in Chinese means to regulate, to cultivate, or to repair. It means to maintain in good condition. This is very different from the religious Daoist Qi training after the Han Dynasty which was called "Lian Qi" (練氣), which is translated "train Qi." "Lian" means to drill or to practice to make stronger.

Many of the Qigong documents written by the Confucians and Daoists were limited to the maintenance of health. The scholar's attitude in Qigong was to follow his natural destiny and maintain his health. This philosophy is quite different from that of the religious Daoist after the Han Dynasty, who believed that one's destiny could be changed. They believed that it is possible to train your Qi to make it stronger; and to extend your life. It is said in scholarly society: "In human life, seventy is rare."[14] You should understand that few of the common people in ancient times lived past seventy because of the lack of good food and modern medical technology. It is also said: "Peace with Heaven and delight in your destiny" (安天樂命); and "Cultivate the body and await destiny" (修身俟命). Compare this with the philosophy of the later Daoists, who said: "One hundred and twenty means dying young."[15] They believed and have proven that human life can be lengthened and destiny can be resisted and overcome.

Confucianism and Daoism were the two major scholarly schools in China, but there were many other schools which were also more or less involved in Qigong practices. We will not discuss them here because there is only a very limited number of Qigong documents from these schools.

Medical Qigong—for Healing. In ancient Chinese society, most emperors respected the scholars and were affected by their philosophy. Doctors were not highly regarded because they made their diagnosis by touching the patient's body, which was considered characteristic of the lower classes in society. Although the doctors developed a profound and successful medical science, they were commonly looked down on by others. However, they continued to work hard and study, and quietly passed down the results of their research to following generations.

Of all the groups studying Qigong in China, the doctors have been at it the longest. Since the discovery of Qi circulation in the human body about four thousand years ago, the Chinese doctors have devoted a major portion of their efforts to studying the behavior of Qi. Their efforts resulted in acupuncture, acupressure or Cavity Press massage, and herbal treatment.

In addition, many Chinese doctors used their medical knowledge to create different sets of Qigong exercises either for maintaining health or for curing specific illnesses. Chinese medical doctors believed that doing only sitting or still meditation to regulate the body, mind, and breathing as the scholars did was not enough to cure sickness. They believed that in order to increase the Qi circulation, you must move. Although a calm and peaceful mind was important for health, exercising the body was more important. They learned through their medical practice that people who exercised properly got sick less often, and their bodies degenerated less quickly than was the case with people who just sat around. They also realized that specific body movements could increase the Qi circulation in specific organs. They reasoned from this that these exercises could also be used to treat specific illnesses and to restore the normal functioning of these organs.

Some of these movements are similar to the way in which certain animals move. It is clear that in order for an animal to survive in the wild, it must have an instinct for how to protect its body. Part of this instinct is concerned with how to build up its Qi, and how to keep its Qi from being lost. We humans have lost many of these instincts over the years that we have been separating ourselves from nature.

Many doctors developed Qigong exercises which were modeled after animal movements to maintain health and cure sickness. A typical and well known set of such exercises is "Wu Qin Xi" (Five Animal Sports)(五禽戲) created by Dr. Jun Qing (君倩). Another famous set based on similar principles is called "Ba Duan Jin" (The Eight Pieces of Brocade)(八段錦). It was created by Marshal Yue Fei (岳飛) who, interestingly enough, was a soldier rather than a doctor.

In addition, using their medical knowledge of Qi circulation, Chinese doctors researched until they found which movements could help cure particular illnesses and health problems. Not surprisingly, many of these movements were not unlike the ones used to maintain health, since many illnesses are caused by unbalanced Qi. When an imbalance continues for a long period of time, the organs will be affected, and may be physically damaged. It is just like running a machine without supplying the proper electrical current—over time, the machine will be damaged. Chinese doctors believe that before physical damage to an organ shows up in a patient's body, there is first an abnormality in the Qi balance and circulation. **Abnormal Qi circulation is the very beginning of illness and organ damage**. When Qi is too positive (Yang) or too negative (Yin) in a specific organ's Qi channel, your physical organ begins to suffer damage. If you do not correct the Qi circulation, that organ will malfunction or degenerate. The best way to heal someone is to adjust and balance the Qi even before there is any physical problem. Therefore, correcting or increasing the normal Qi circulation is the major goal of acupuncture or acupressure treatments. Herbs and special diets are also considered important treatments in regulating the Qi in the body.

As long as the illness is limited to the level of Qi stagnation and there is no physical organ damage, the Qigong exercises used for maintaining health can be used to readjust the Qi circulation and treat the problem. However, if the sickness is already so serious that the physical organs have started to fail, then the situation has become critical and a specific treatment is necessary. The treatment can be acupuncture, herbs, or even an operation, as well as specific Qigong exercises designed to speed up the healing or even to cure the sickness. For example, ulcers and asthma can often be cured or helped by some simple exercises. Recently in both mainland China and Taiwan, certain Qigong exercises have been shown to be effective in treating certain kinds of cancer.

Over the thousands of years of observing nature and themselves, some Qigong practitioners went even deeper. They realized that the body's Qi circulation changes with the seasons, and that it is a good idea to help the body out during these periodic adjustments. They noticed also that in each season different organs have characteristic problems. For example, in the beginning of autumn the lungs have to adapt to the colder air that you are breathing. While this adjustment is going on, the lungs are susceptible to disturbance, so your lungs may feel uncomfortable and you may catch colds easily. Your digestive system is also affected during seasonal changes. Your appetite may increase, or you may have diarrhea. When the temperature goes down, your kidneys and bladder will start to give you trouble. For example, because the kidneys are stressed, you may feel pain in the back. Focusing on these seasonal Qi disorders, the meditators created a set of movements which can be used to speed up the body's adjustment.

In addition to Marshal Yue Fei, many people who were not doctors also created sets of medical Qigong. These sets were probably originally created to maintain health, and later were also used for curing sickness.

Martial Qigong—for Fighting. Chinese martial Qigong was probably not developed until Da Mo wrote the *Muscle/Tendon Changing Classic* in the Shaolin Temple during the Liang Dynasty (502-557 A.D.). When Shaolin monks trained Da Mo's Muscle/Tendon Changing Qigong, they found that they could not only improve their health but also greatly increase the power of their martial techniques. Since then, many martial styles have developed Qigong sets to increase their effectiveness. In addition, many martial styles have been created based on Qigong theory. Martial artists have played a major role in Chinese Qigong society.

When Qigong theory was first applied to the martial arts, it was used to increase the power and efficiency of the muscles. The theory is very simple—**the mind (Yi) is used to lead Qi to the muscles to energize them so that they function more efficiently**. The average person generally uses his muscles at about 40 percent maximum efficiency. If one can train his concentration and use his strong Yi (the mind generated from clear thinking) to lead Qi to the muscles effectively, he will be able to energize the muscles to a higher level and, therefore, increase his fighting effectiveness.

As acupuncture theory became better understood, fighting techniques were able to reach even more advanced levels. Martial artists learned to attack specific areas, such as vital acupuncture cavities, to disturb the enemy's Qi flow and create imbalances which caused injury or even death. In order to do this, the practitioner must understand the route and timing of the Qi circulation in the human body. He also has to train so that he can strike the cavities accurately and to the correct depth. These cavity strike techniques are called "Dian Xue" (點穴)(Pointing Cavities) or "Dian Mai" (點脈)(Pointing Vessels).

Most of the martial Qigong practices help to improve the practitioner's health. However, there are other martial Qigong practices which, although they build up some special skill which is useful for fighting, also damage the practitioner's health. An example of this is Iron Sand Palm (Tie Sha Zhang, 鐵砂掌). Although this training can build up amazing destructive power, it can also harm your hands and affect the Qi circulation in the hands and internal organs.

As mentioned earlier, since the 6th century, many martial styles have been created which were based on Qigong theory. They can be roughly divided into external and internal styles.

The external styles emphasize building Qi in the limbs to coordinate with the physical martial techniques. They follow the theory of Wai Dan (External Elixir) Qigong, which usually generates Qi in the limbs through special exercises. The concentrated mind is used during the exercises to energize the Qi. This increases muscular strength significantly, and therefore increases the effectiveness of the martial techniques. Qigong can also be used to train the body to resist punches and kicks. In this training, Qi is led to energize the skin and the muscles, enabling them to resist a blow without injury. This training is commonly called "Iron Shirt" (Tie Bu Shan, 鐵布衫) or "Golden Bell Cover" (Jin Zhong Zhao, 金鐘罩). The martial styles which use Wai Dan Qigong training are normally called external styles (Wai Jia, 外家) or Hard Qigong training is called Hard Gong (Ying Gong, 硬功). Shaolin Gongfu is a typical example of a style which uses Wai Dan martial Qigong.

Although Wai Dan Qigong can help the martial artist increase his power, there is a disadvantage. Because Wai Dan Qigong emphasizes training the external muscles, it can cause over-development. This can cause a problem called "energy dispersion" (San Gong, 散功) when the practitioner gets older. In order to remedy this, when an external martial artist reaches a high level of external Qigong training he will start training internal Qigong, which specializes in curing the energy dispersion problem. That is why it is said: "Shaolin Gongfu from external to internal."

Internal Martial Qigong is based on the theory of Nei Dan (Internal Elixir). In this method, Qi is generated in the body instead of the limbs, and this Qi is then led to the limbs to increase power. In order to lead Qi to the limbs, the techniques must be soft and muscle usage must be kept to a minimum. The training and theory of Nei Dan martial Qigong is much more difficult than those of Wai Dan martial Qigong. Interested readers should refer to the book: *Advanced Yang Style Tai Chi Chuan—Tai Chi Theory and Tai Chi Jing*, available from YMAA Publication Center.

Several internal martial styles were created in the Wudang (武當山) and Emei Mountains (峨嵋山). Popular styles are Taijiquan, Baguazhang, Liu He Ba Fa, and Xingyiquan. However, you should understand that even the internal martial styles, which are commonly called Soft Styles, must on some occasions use muscular strength while fighting. That means in order to have strong power in the fight, the Qi must be led to the muscular body and manifested externally. Therefore, once an internal martial artist has achieved a degree of competence in internal Qigong, he or she should also learn how to use harder, more external techniques. That is why it is said: "The internal styles are from soft to hard."

In the last fifty years, some of the Taiji Qigong or Taijiquan practitioners have developed training which is mainly for health, and is called "Wuji Qigong" (無極氣功), which means "no extremities Qigong." Wuji is the state of neutrality which precedes Taiji, which is the state of relative, complimentary opposites. When there are thoughts and feeling in your mind, there is Yin and Yang, but if you can still your mind you can return to the emptiness of Wuji. When you achieve this state your mind is centered and clear, your body relaxed, and your Qi is able to flow naturally and smoothly to reach the proper balance by itself. Wuji Qigong has become very popular in many parts of China, especially Shanghai and Canton.

You can see that, although Qigong is widely studied in Chinese martial society, originally the main focus of training was on increasing fighting ability rather than health. Good health was considered a by-product of training. It was not until this century that the health aspect of martial Qigong started receiving greater attention. This is especially true in the internal martial arts.

Religious Qigong—for Enlightenment or Buddhahood. Religious Qigong, though not as popular as other categories in China, is recognized as having achieved the highest accomplishments of all the Qigong categories. It used to be kept secret in the monastic society, and it is only in this century that it has been revealed to laymen.

In China, religious Qigong includes mainly Daoist and Buddhist Qigong. The main purpose of their training is striving for enlightenment, or what the Buddhists refer to as Buddhahood. They are looking for a way to lift themselves above normal human suffering, and to escape from the cycle of continual reincarnation. They believe that all human suffering is caused by the seven emotions and six desires (Qi Qing Liu Yu, 七情六慾). The seven emotions are **happiness** (Xi, 喜), **anger** (Nu, 怒), **sorrow** (Ai, 哀), **joy** (Le, 樂), **love** (Ai, 愛), **hate** (Hen, 恨), and **desire** (Yu, 慾). The six desires are the six sensory pleasures derived from the eyes, ears, nose, tongue, body, and mind. If you are still bound to these emotions and desires, you will reincarnate after your death. To avoid reincarnation, you must train your spirit to reach a very high stage where it is strong enough to be independent after your death. This spirit will enter the heavenly kingdom and gain eternal peace. This training is hard to do in the everyday world, so practitioners frequently flee society and move into the solitude of the mountains, where they can concentrate all of their energies on self-cultivation.

Religious Qigong practitioners train to strengthen their internal Qi to nourish their spirit (Shen) until the spirit is able to survive the death of the physical body. Marrow/Brain Washing Qigong training is necessary to reach this stage. It enables them to lead Qi to the forehead, where the spirit resides, and raise the brain to a higher energy state. This training used to be restricted to only a few priests who had reached an advanced level. Tibetan Buddhists were also heavily involved in this training. Over the last two thousand years the Tibetan Buddhists, the Chinese Buddhists, and the Daoists have followed the same principles to become the three major religious schools of Qigong training.

This religious striving toward enlightenment or Buddhahood is recognized as the highest and most difficult level of Qigong. Many Qigong practitioners reject the rigors of this religious striving, and practice Marrow/Brain Washing Qigong solely for the purpose of longevity. It was these people who eventually revealed the secrets of Marrow/Brain Washing to the outside world. If you are interested in knowing more about this training, you may refer to: *Muscle/Tendon Changing and Marrow/Brain Washing Chi Kung* available from YMAA Publication Center.

From the above brief summary, you may obtain a general concept of how Chinese Qigong can be categorized. From the understanding of this general concept, you should not have further doubt about any Qigong you are training.

In the next section, we will discuss general Qigong training theory. This theoretical discussion of Qigong practice will offer you a foundation upon which to build your training. Without this scientific theoretical support, your mind will continue wondering and wandering. Understanding the theory is like learning how to read a map, which can direct you to the final goal of practice without confusion.

1-5. Qigong Training Theory

Many people think that Qigong is a difficult subject to comprehend. In some ways, this is true. However, you must understand one thing: regardless of how difficult the Qigong theory and practice of a particular style is, the basic theory and principles are very simple and remain the same for all Qigong styles. The basic theory and principles are the root of the entire Qigong practice. If you understand these roots, you will be able to grasp the key to the practice and grow. All of the Qigong styles originated from these roots, but each one has blossomed differently.

In this section we will discuss these basic Qigong training theories and principles. With this knowledge as foundation, you will be able to understand not only what you should be doing, but also why you are doing it. Naturally, it is impossible to discuss all of the basic Qigong ideas in such a short section. However, it will offer you the key to open the gate into the spacious, four thousand year old garden of Chinese Qigong. If you wish to know more about the theory of Qigong, please refer to *The Root of Chinese Qigong*.

The Concept of Yin and Yang, Kan and Li

The concept of Yin (陰) and Yang (陽) is the foundation of Chinese philosophy. From this philosophy, Chinese culture was developed. Naturally, this includes Chinese medicine and Qigong practice. Therefore, in order to understand Qigong, first you should study the concept of Yin and Yang. In addition, you should also understand the concept of Kan (坎) and Li (離) which, unfortunately, has been commonly confused with the concept of Yin and Yang even in China.

The Chinese have long believed that the universe is made up of two opposite forces—Yin and Yang—which must balance each other. When these two forces begin to lose their balance, nature finds a way to re-balance them. If the imbalance is significant, disaster will occur. However, when these two forces interact with each other smoothly and harmoniously, they manifest power and generate the millions of living things.

As mentioned earlier, Yin and Yang theory is also applied to the three great natural powers: Heaven, Earth, and Man. For example, if the Yin and Yang forces of Heaven (i.e., energy which comes to us from the sky) lose their balance, there can be tornadoes, hurricanes, or other natural disasters. When the Yin and Yang forces lose their balance on earth, rivers can change their paths and earthquakes can occur. When the Yin and Yang forces in the human body lose their balance, sickness and even death can occur. Experience has shown that the Yin and Yang balance in man is affected by the Yin and Yang balances of the earth and heaven. Similarly, the Yin and Yang balance of the earth is influenced by the heaven's Yin and Yang. Therefore, if you wish to have a healthy body and live a long life, you need to know how to adjust your body's Yin and Yang, and how to coordinate your Qi with the Yin and Yang energy of heaven and earth. The study of Yin and Yang in the human body is the root of Chinese medicine and Qigong.

Furthermore, the Chinese have also classified everything in the universe according to Yin and Yang. Even feelings, thoughts, strategy and the spirit are covered. For example, female is Yin and male is Yang, night is Yin and day is Yang, weak is Yin and strong is Yang, backward is Yin and forward is Yang, sad is Yin and happy is Yang, defense is Yin and offense is Yang, and so on.

Practitioners of Chinese medicine and Qigong believe that they must seek to understand the Yin and Yang of nature and the human body before they can adjust and regulate the body's energy balance into a more harmonious state. Only then can health be maintained and the causes of sicknesses be corrected.

Another thing which you should understand is that the concept of Yin and Yang is relative instead of absolute. For example, the number seven is Yang compared with three. However, if seven is compared with ten, then it is Yin. That means in order to decide Yin or Yang, a reference point must first be chosen. Therefore, if five is the Yin and Yang balance number, then seven is Yang and three is Yin. If we choose zero as the Yin and Yang balance number, then any positive number is Yang and any negative number is Yin.

However, if what we are interested in is the most negative number, then we may choose the negative number as Yang and positive number as Yin with zero as the central number. For example, generally speaking in Qigong, techniques that can be seen physically and are the manifestation of Qi are considered Yang, and the techniques that cannot be seen but felt are considered Yin. When the Yin and Yang concept is applied in Chinese medicine, since the Qi is the major concern and plays the main role in medicine, it is considered Yang, while the blood (physical) is considered Yin.

Now let us discuss how the concept of Yin and Yang is applied to the Qi circulating in the human body. Many people, even some Qigong practitioners, are still confused by this. When it is said that Qi can be either Yin or Yang, it does not mean that there are two different kinds of Qi like male and female, fire and water, or positive and negative charges. Qi is energy, and energy itself does not have Yin and Yang. It is like the energy which is generated from the sparking of negative and positive charges. Charges have the potential for generating energy, but are not the energy itself.

When it is said that Qi is Yin or Yang, it means that the Qi is too strong or too weak for a particular circumstance. Again, it is relative and not absolute. Naturally, this implies that the potential which generates the Qi is strong or weak. For example, the Qi from the sun is Yang Qi, and Qi from the moon is Yin Qi. This is because the sun's energy is Yang in comparison to Human Qi, while the moon's is Yin. In any discussion of energy where people are involved, Human Qi is used as the standard. People are always especially interested in what concerns them directly, so it is natural that we are interested primarily in Human Qi and tend to view all Qi from the perspective of Human Qi. This is not unlike looking at the universe from the physical perspective of the Earth.

When we look at the Yin and Yang of Qi within the human body, however, we must redefine our point of reference. For example, when a person is dead, his residual Human Qi (Gui Qi or ghost Qi, 鬼氣) is weak compared to a living person's. Therefore, the ghost Qi is Yin as it dissipates, while the living person's Qi is Yang. When discussing Qi within the body, in the Lung Channel for example, the reference point is the normal, healthy status of the Qi there. If the Qi is stronger than it is in the normal state, it is Yang, and, naturally, if it is weaker than this, it is Yin. There are twelve parts of the human body that are considered organs in Chinese medicine, six of them are Yin and six are Yang. The Yin organs are the **Heart**, **Lungs**, **Kidneys**, **Liver**, **Spleen**, and **Pericardium**, and the Yang organs are the **Large Intestine**, **Small Intestine**, **Stomach**, **Gall Bladder**, **Urinary Bladder**, and **Triple Burner**. Generally speaking, the Qi level of the Yin organs is lower than that of the Yang organs. The Yin organs store Original Essence and process the Essence obtained from food and air, while the Yang organs handle digestion and excretion.

When the Qi in any of your organs is not in its normal state, you feel uncomfortable. If it is very much off from the normal state, the organ will start to malfunction and you may become sick. When this happens, the Qi in your entire body will also be affected and you will feel too Yang, perhaps feverish, or too Yin, such as the weakness after diarrhea.

Your body's Qi level is also affected by your natural environment, such as the weather, climate, and seasonal changes. Therefore, when the body's Qi level is classified, the reference point is the level which feels most comfortable for those particular circumstances. Naturally, each of us is a little bit different, and what feels best and most natural for one person may be a bit different from what is right for another person. That is why the doctor will usually ask "How do you feel?" It is according to your own standard that you are judged.

Breathing is closely related to the state of your Qi, and is therefore also considered Yin or Yang. When you exhale you expel air from your lungs, your mind moves outward, and the Qi around the body expands. In the Chinese martial arts, the exhale is generally used to expand the Qi to energize the muscles during an attack. Therefore, you can see that the exhale is Yang—it is expanding, offensive, and strong. Naturally, based on the same theory, the inhale is considered Yin.

Your breathing is closely related to your emotions. When you lose your temper, your breathing is short and fast, i.e., Yang. When you are sad, your body is more Yin, and you inhale more than you exhale in order to absorb Qi from the air to balance the body's Yin and bring the body back into balance. When you are excited and happy your body is Yang, and your exhale is longer than your inhale to get rid of the excess Yang which is caused by the excitement.

As mentioned before, your mind is also closely related to your Qi. Therefore, when your Qi is Yang, your mind is usually also Yang (excited) and vice versa. The mind can also be classified according to the Qi which generated it. The mind (Yi) which is generated from the calm and peaceful Qi obtained from the Original Essence is considered Yin. The mind (Xin) which originates with the food and air Essence is emotional, scattered, and excited, and it is considered Yang. The spirit, which is related to the Qi, can also be classified as Yang or Yin based on its origin.

Do not confuse Yin Qi and Yang Qi with Fire Qi and Water Qi. When the Yin and Yang of Qi are mentioned, it refers to the level of Qi according to some reference point. However, when Water and Fire Qi are mentioned, it refers to the quality of the Qi. If you are interested in reading more about the Yin and Yang of Qi, please refer to the books: *The Root of Chinese Qigong* and *Muscle/Tendon Changing and Marrow/Brain Washing Chi Kung*, from YMAA Publication Center.

The terms **Kan** and **Li** occur frequently in Qigong documents. In the Eight Trigrams Kan represents "Water" while Li represents "Fire." However, the everyday terms for water and fire are also often used. Kan and Li training has long been of major importance to Qigong practitioners. In order to understand why, you must understand these two words, and the theory behind them.

First you should understand that though Kan-Li and Yin-Yang are related, Kan and Li are not Yin and Yang. **Kan is Water, which is able to cool your body down and make it more Yin, while Li is Fire, which warms your body and makes it more Yang. Kan and Li are the methods or causes, while Yin and Yang are the results**. When Kan and Li are adjusted and regulated correctly, Yin and Yang will be balanced and interact harmoniously.

Qigong practitioners believe that your body is always too Yang, unless you are sick or have not eaten for a long time, in which case your body may be more Yin. Since your body is always Yang, it is degenerating and burning out. It is believed that this is the cause of aging. If you can use Water to cool down your body, you will be able to slow down the degeneration process and thereby lengthen your life. This is the main reason why **Chinese Qigong practitioners have been studying ways of improving the quality of the Water in their bodies, and of reducing the quantity of the Fire**. I believe that as a Qigong practitioner you should always keep this subject at the top of your list for study and research. If you earnestly ponder and experiment, you will be able to grasp the trick of adjusting them.

If you want to learn how to adjust them, you must understand that Water and Fire mean many things in your body. The first concerns your Qi. As mentioned earlier, Qi is classified as Fire and Water. When your Qi is not pure and causes your physical body to heat up and your mental/spiritual body to become unstable (Yang), it is classified as Fire Qi. The Qi which is pure and is able to cool both your physical and spiritual bodies (make them more Yin) is considered Water Qi. However, you body can never be purely Water. Water can cool down the Fire, but it must never totally quench it, because then you would be dead. It is also said that Fire Qi is able to agitate and stimulate the emotions, and from these emotions generate a "mind." This mind is called Xin (心), and is considered the Fire mind, Yang mind, or emotional mind. On the other hand, the mind that Water Qi generates is calm, steady, and wise. This mind is called Yi (意), and is considered to be the Water mind or wisdom mind. If your spirit is nourished by the Fire Qi, although your spirit may be high, it will be scattered and confused (a Yang spirit). Naturally, if the spirit is nourished and raised up by Water Qi, it will be firm and steady (a Yin mind). When your Yi is able to govern your emotional Xin effectively, your will (strong emotional intention) can be firm.

You can see from this discussion that your Qi is the main cause of the Yin and Yang of your physical body, your mind, and your spirit. To regulate your body's Yin and Yang, you must learn how to regulate your body's Water and Fire Qi, but in order to do this efficiently you must know their sources.

Once you have grasped the concepts of Yin-Yang and Kan-Li, then you have to think about how to adjust Kan and Li so that you can balance the Yin and Yang in your body.

Theoretically, a Qigong practitioner would like to keep his body in a state of Yin-Yang balance, which means the "center" point of the Yin and Yang forces. This center point is commonly called "Wuji" (無極)(no extremities). It is believed that Wuji is the original, natural state where Yin and Yang are not distinguished. In the Wuji state, nature is peaceful and calm. In the Wuji state, all of the Yin and Yang forces have gradually combined harmoniously and disappeared. When this Wuji theory is applied to human beings, it is the final goal of Qigong practice where your mind is neutral and absolutely calm. The Wuji state makes it possible for you to find the origin of your life, and to combine your Qi with the Qi of nature.

The ultimate goal and purpose of Qigong practice is to find this peaceful and natural state. In order to reach this goal, you must first understand your body's Yin and Yang so that you can balance them by adjusting your Kan and Li. Only when your Yin and Yang are balanced will you be able to find the center balance point, the Wuji state.

Theoretically, between the two extremes of Yin and Yang are millions of paths (i.e., different Kan and Li methods) which can lead you to the neutral center. This accounts for the hundreds of different styles of Qigong which have been created over the years. You can see that the theory of Yin and Yang and the methods of Kan and Li are the root of training all Chinese Qigong styles. Without this root, the essence of Qigong practice would be lost.

Three Treasures—Jing, Qi, and Shen (三寶-精、氣、神)

Before you start any Qigong training you must also understand the three treasures of your body (San Bao, 三寶): **Jing** (Essence, 精), **Qi** (Internal Energy, 氣), and **Shen** (Spirit, 神). They are also called the three origins or the three roots (San Yuan, 三元), because they are considered the origins and roots of your life. Jing means

Essence, the most original and refined part. Jing is the original source and most basic part of every living thing, and determines its nature and characteristics. It is the root of life. Sperm is called Jing Zi (精子), which means "Essence of the Son," because it contains the Jing of the father which is passed on to his son (or daughter) and becomes the child's Jing.

Qi, known as bioelectricity today, is the internal energy of your body. It is like the electricity which passes through a machine to keep it running. Qi comes either from the conversion of the Jing which you have received from your parents, or from the food you eat and the air you breathe.

Shen is the center of your mind and being. It is what makes you human, because animals do not have a Shen. The Shen in your body must be nourished by your Qi or energy. When your Qi is full, your Shen will be enlivened.

Chinese meditators and Qigong practitioners believe that the body contains two general types of Qi. The first type is called **Pre-Birth Qi** or **Pre-Heaven Qi** (Xian Tian Qi, 先天氣), and it comes from converted Original Jing (Yuan Jing, 元精), which you get from your parents at conception. The second type, which is called **Post-Birth Qi** or **Post Heaven Qi** (Hou Tian Qi, 後天氣), is drawn from the Jing of our food and air intake. When this Qi flows or is led to the brain, it can energize the Shen and soul. This energized and raised Shen is able to govern and lead the Qi to the entire body.

Each one of these three elements or treasures has its own root. You must know the roots so that you can strengthen and protect your three treasures.

1. Your body requires many kinds of Jing. Except for the Jing which you inherit from your parents, which is called Original Jing (Yuan Jing, 元精), all other Jings must be obtained from food and air. Among all of these Jings, Original Jing is the most important one. It is the root and the seed of your life, and your basic strength. If your parents were strong and healthy, your Original Jing will be strong and healthy, and you will have a strong foundation on which to grow. The Chinese people believe that in order to stay healthy and live a long life, you must protect and maintain this Jing.

    According to Chinese medicine, the root of Original Jing before your birth was in your parents. After birth this Original Jing stays in its residence—the kidneys, which are considered the root of your Jing. When you keep this root strong, you will have sufficient Original Jing to supply to your body. Although you cannot increase the amount of Original Jing you have, Qigong training can improve the quality of your Jing. Qigong can also teach you how to convert your Jing into Original Qi more efficiently, and how to use this Qi effectively.

    If we analyze the concept of Jing from a modern physical scientific point of view, we might postulate that Jing is in the genetic material which we inherited from our parents. From this material, the structure and health of one person is different from all others. From different genes, the different levels of hormones in different people are controlled. When Chinese medicine says that the Original Jing is stored in the kidneys, it implies the hormones which are produced in the adrenal glands. According to Chinese medicine, there is no record of the endocrine glands. This implies that Chinese medicine has never understood the function of the endocrine. In my opinion, the Jing (essence) is stored in all of the endocrine glands. I believe that the most significant gland which stores the essence and affects the level of the entire body's Jing (hormone production) is the pituitary gland (corresponding to the Upper Dan Tian).

2. According to Chinese medicine and Qigong, Qi is converted both from the Jing which you have inherited from your parents and from the Jing which you draw from the food and air you breathe. Qi that is converted from the Original Jing which you inherited is called Original Qi (Yuan Qi, 元氣).[16] Just as Original Jing is the most important type of Jing, Original Qi is the most important type of Qi. It is pure and of high quality, while the Qi from food and air may make your body too positive or too negative, depending on how and where you absorb it. When you retain and protect your Original Jing, you will be able to generate Original Qi in a pure, continuous stream. As a Qigong practitioner, you must know how to convert your Original Jing into Original Qi in a smooth, steady stream.

Since your Original Qi comes from your Original Jing, they both have the kidneys for their root. When your kidneys are strong, the Original Jing is strong, and the Original Qi converted from this Original Jing will also be full and strong. This Qi resides in the Lower Dan Tian in your abdomen. Once you learn how to convert your Original Jing, you will be able to supply your body with all the Qi it needs.

Again, if we analyze the above concepts, we can see that the essence here means the hormone level which is produced from the adrenal glands on the top of your kidneys. In fact, we have already seen that the pituitary gland is considered the master of the glands, and when the hormone production in this gland is high, the hormone production of all other Endocrine Glands will also be high. When the hormone level of the body is high, the Qi is abundant and the circulation is smooth. When the hormone production level is high in the pituitary gland, the spirit (Shen, 神) residing in the center of your brain will be high. When the spirit is high, it is able to strongly and smoothly direct the Qi circulating in the body for function, repair and healing. This results in the development of spiritual healing science.

3. Shen (i.e., spirit, 神) is the force which keeps you alive. It has no substance, but it gives expression and appearance to your Jing. Shen is also the control tower for the Qi. When your Shen is strong, your Qi is strong and you can lead it efficiently. The root of Shen (Spirit) is your mind (Yi, or intention). When your brain is energized and stimulated, your mind will be more aware and you will be able to concentrate more intensely. Also, your Shen will be raised.

Advanced Qigong practitioners believe that your brain must always be sufficiently nourished by your Qi. It is the Qi which keeps your mind clear and concentrated. With an abundant Qi supply, the mind can be energized, and can raise the Shen and enhance your vitality.

The deeper levels of Qigong training include the conversion of Jing into Qi (Lian Jing Hua Qi, 練精化氣), which is then led to the brain to raise the Shen (Lian Qi Hua Shen, 練氣化神). This process is called "Huan Jing Bu Nao" (還精補腦) and means "return the Jing to nourish the brain." When Qi is led to the head, it stays at the Upper Dan Tian (at the center of the forehead), which is the residence of your Shen. Qi and Shen are mutually related. When your Shen is weak, your Qi is weak, and your body will degenerate rapidly. Shen is the headquarters of Qi. Likewise, Qi supports the Shen, energizing it and keeping it sharp, clear, and strong. If the Qi in your body is weak, your Shen will also be weak.

Scientifically, in order to maintain a high hormone production level, you must continue to supply bioelectricity to the pituitary gland. Without this basic energy, the gland will function inadequately. Therefore, one of the main Qigong practices is learning, through meditation, how to lead the Qi to the brain and nourish the pituitary gland.

From the above discussion, you can see that in order to have a healthy and strong body, you must first learn how to keep the Yin and Yang balanced in your body. In addition, you should also learn how to adjust or regulate your body, allowing you to fit in the natural environment more harmoniously. Furthermore, you should learn how to **retain and generate your Jing, strengthen and smooth your Qi flow**, and **enlighten your Shen**. That means you should learn how to maintain the hormone production of your body, how to store the Qi in your Lower Dan Tian (battery) and smoothly circulate it in your body, and how to lead the Qi to the brain to nourish your Spirit. If you are interested in the further pursuit of enlightenment, then you must learn how to regulate your mind to a neutral state and build up a Spiritual Embryo (Sheng Tai, 聖胎). From the cultivation of this spiritual embryo, you will be able to separate your spiritual body and your physical body. If you are interested in this subject, please refer to *Muscle/Tendon Changing and Marrow/Brain Washing Chi Kung*, from YMAA Publication Center.

Qigong Training Theory

Every Qigong form or practice has its special training purpose and theory. If you do not know the purpose and theory, you have lost the root (meaning) of the practice. Therefore, as a Qigong practitioner, you must continue to ponder and practice until you understand the root of every set or form.

Now that you have learned the basic theory of the Qigong practice, let us discuss the general training principles. In Chinese Qigong society, it is commonly known that in order to reach the goal of Qigong practice, you must learn how to **regulate the body** (Tiao Shen, 調身), **regulate the breathing** (Tiao Xi, 調息), **regulate the emo-**

tional mind (Tiao Xin, 調心), **regulate the Qi** (Tiao Qi, 調氣), and **regulate the spirit** (Tiao Shen, 調神). Tiao in Chinese is constructed from two words; 言 (Yan, means speaking or talking) and 周 (Zhou, means round or complete). That means the roundness (i.e., harmony) or the completeness is accomplished by negotiation. Like an out of tune piano, you must adjust it and make it harmonious. This implies that, when you are regulating one of the above five processes, you must also coordinate and harmonize the other four regulating elements.

Regulating the body includes understanding how to find and build the root of the body, as well as the root of the individual forms you are practicing. To build a firm root, you must know how to keep your center, how to balance your body, and most important of all, how to relax so that the Qi can flow.

To regulate your breathing, you must learn how to breathe so that your respiration and your mind mutually correspond and cooperate. When you breathe this way, your mind will be able to attain peace more quickly, and therefore concentrate more easily on leading the Qi.

Regulating the mind involves learning how to keep your mind calm, peaceful, and centered, so that you can judge situations objectively and lead Qi to the desired places. The mind is the main key to success in Qigong practice.

Regulating the Qi is one of the ultimate goals of Qigong practice. In order to regulate your Qi effectively you must first have regulated your body, breathing, and mind. Only then will your mind be clear enough to sense how the Qi is distributed in your body, and understand how to adjust it.

For Buddhist and Daoist priests, who seek enlightenment or Buddhahood, regulating the spirit (Shen) is the final goal of Qigong. This enables them to maintain a neutral, objective perspective of life, and this perspective is the eternal life of the Buddha. The average Qigong practitioner has lower goals. He raises his spirit in order to increase his concentration and enhance his vitality. This makes it possible for him to lead Qi effectively throughout his entire body so that it carries out the managing and guarding duties. This maintains health and slows the aging process.

If you understand these few things you will be able to quickly enter into the field of Qigong. Without all of these important elements, your training will be ineffective and your time will be wasted.

Before you start training, you must first understand that all of the training originates in your mind. You must have a clear idea of what you are doing, and your mind must be calm, centered, and balanced, This also implies that your feeling, sensing, and judgment must be objective and accurate, requiring emotional balance and a clear mind. This takes a lot of hard work, but once you have reached this level you will have built the root of your physical training, and your Yi (mind) will be able to lead your Qi throughout your physical body.

Regulating the Body (Tiao Shen, 調身)

When you learn any Qigong, either moving or still, the first step is to learn the correct postures or movements. After you have learned the postures and movements, learn how to improve them until you can perform the forms accurately. Then, you start to regulate your body until it has reached the stage that provides the best condition for the Qi to build up or to circulate.

In Still Qigong practice or Soft Qigong movement, you must to adjust your body until it is in the most **comfortable** and **relaxed** state. This implies that your body must be centered and balanced. If it is not, you will be tense and uneasy, and this will affect the judgment of your Yi and the circulation of your Qi. In Chinese medical society it is said: "(When) shape (body's posture) is not correct, then the Qi will not be smooth. (When) the Qi is not smooth, the Yi (wisdom mind) will not be peaceful. (When) the Yi is not peaceful, then the Qi is disordered."[17] You should understand that the relaxation of your body originates with your Yi. Therefore, before you can relax your body, you must first relax or regulate your mind (Yi). This is called "Shen Xin Ping Heng" (身心平衡), which means "Body and heart (i.e., mind) balanced." The body and the mind are mutually related. A relaxed and balanced body helps your Yi to relax and concentrate. When your Yi is at peace and can judge things accurately, your body will be relaxed, balanced, centered, and rooted. Only when you are rooted, then you will be able to raise your spirit of vitality.

Relaxation. Relaxation is one of the major keys to success in Qigong. You should remember that **only when you are relaxed will all your Qi channels be open**. In order to be relaxed, your Yi must first be relaxed and calm. When the Yi coordinates with your breathing, your body will be able to relax.

In Qigong practice there are three levels of relaxation. The first level is the external physical relaxation, or postural relaxation. This is a very superficial level, and almost anyone can reach it. It consists of adopting a comfortable stance and avoiding unnecessary strain in how you stand and move. The second level is the relaxation of the muscles and tendons. To do this your Yi must be directed deep into the muscles and tendons. This relaxation will help open your Qi channels, and will allow the Qi to sink and accumulate in the Dan Tian.

The final stage is the relaxation which reaches the internal organs and the bone marrow. Remember, **only if you can relax deep into your body will your mind be able to lead the Qi there**. Only at this stage will the Qi be able to reach everywhere. Then you will feel transparent—as if your whole body had disappeared. If you can reach this level of relaxation, you will be able to communicate with your organs and use Qigong to adjust or regulate the Qi disorders that are giving you problems. You will also be able to protect your organs more effectively, and therefore slow down their degeneration.

Rooting. In all Qigong practice it is very important to be rooted. Being rooted means to be stable and in firm contact with the ground. If you want to push a car, you have to be rooted so the force you exert into the car will be balanced by a force into the ground. If you are not rooted, when you push the car you will only push yourself away, and not move the car. Your root is made up of your body's root, center, and balance.

Before you can develop your root, you must first relax and let your body "settle." As you relax, the tension in the various parts of your body will dissolve, and you will find a comfortable way to stand. You will stop fighting the ground to keep your body up, and will learn to rely on your body's structure to support itself. This lets the muscles relax even more. Since your body isn't struggling to stand up, your Yi won't be pushing upward, and your body, mind, and Qi will all be able to sink. If you let dirty water sit quietly, the impurities will gradually settle down to the bottom, leaving the water above it clear. In the same way, if you relax your body enough to let it settle, your Qi will sink to your Dan Tian and the Bubbling Wells (Yongquan, K-1, 湧泉) in your feet, and your mind will become clear. Then you can begin to develop your root.

To root your body you must imitate a tree and grow an invisible root under your feet. This will give you a firm root to keep you stable in your training. **Your root must be wide as well as deep**. Naturally, your Yi must grow first, because it is the Yi which leads the Qi. Your Yi must be able to lead the Qi to your feet, and be able to communicate with the ground. Only when your Yi can communicate with the ground will your Qi be able to grow beyond your feet and enter the ground to build the root. The Bubbling Well cavity is the gate which enables your Qi to communicate with the ground.

After you have gained your root, you must learn how to keep your center. A stable center will make your Qi develop evenly and uniformly. If you lose this center, your Qi will not be led evenly. In order to keep your body centered, you must first center your Yi, and then match your body to it. Only under these conditions will the Qigong forms you practice have their root. Your mental and physical centers are the keys which enable you to lead your Qi beyond your body.

Balance is the product of rooting and centering. Balance includes balancing the Qi and the physical body. It does not matter which aspect of balance you are dealing with, first you must balance your Yi, and only then can you balance your Qi and your physical body. If your Yi is balanced, it can help you to make accurate judgments, and therefore to correct the path of the Qi flow.

Rooting includes not just rooting the body, but also the form or movement. The root of any form or movement is found in its purpose or principle. For example, in certain Qigong exercises you want to lead the Qi to your palms. In order to do this you may imagine that you are pushing an object forward while keeping your muscles relaxed. In this exercise, your elbows must be down to build the sense of root for the push. If you raise the elbows, you lose the sense of "intention" of the movement, because the push would be ineffective if you were pushing something for real. Since the intention or purpose of the movement is its reason for being, you now have a purposeless movement, and you have no reason to lead Qi in any particular way. Therefore, in this case, the elbow is the root of the movement.

Regulating the Breath (Tiao Xi, 調息)

Regulating the breath means to regulate your breathing until it is calm, smooth, and peaceful. Only when you have reached this point will you be able to make the breathing **deep**, **slender**, **long**, and **soft**, which is required for successful Qigong practice.

Breathing is affected by your emotions. For example, when you are angry or excited you exhale more strongly than you inhale. When you are sad, you inhale more strongly than you exhale. When your mind is peaceful and calm, your inhalation and exhalation are relatively equal. In order to keep your breathing calm, peaceful, and steady, your mind and emotions must first be calm and neutral. Therefore, in order to regulate your breathing, you must first regulate your mind.

The other side of the coin is that you can use your breathing to control your Yi. When your breathing is uniform, it is as if you were hypnotizing your Yi, which helps to calm it. You can see that Yi and breathing are interdependent, and that they cooperate with each other. Deep and calm breathing relaxes you and keeps your mind clear. It fills your lungs with plenty of air, so that your brain and entire body have an adequate supply of oxygen. In addition, deep and complete breathing enables the diaphragm to move up and down, which massages and stimulates the internal organs. For this reason, deep breathing exercises are also called "internal organ exercises."

Deep and complete breathing does not mean that you inhale and exhale to the maximum. This would cause the lungs and the surrounding muscles to tense up, which in turn would keep the air from circulating freely, and hinder the absorption of oxygen. Without enough oxygen, your mind becomes scattered, and the rest of your body tenses up. In correct breathing, you inhale and exhale to about 70 percent or 80 percent of capacity, so that your lungs stay relaxed.

You can conduct an easy experiment. Inhale deeply so that your lungs are completely full, and time how long you can hold your breath. Then try inhaling to only about 70 percent of your capacity, and see how long you can hold your breath. You will find that with the latter method you can last much longer than the first one. This is simply because the lungs and the surrounding muscles are relaxed. When they are relaxed, the rest of your body and your mind can also relax, which significantly decreases your need for oxygen. Therefore, when you regulate your breathing, the first priority is to keep your lungs relaxed and calm.

When training, your mind must first be calm so that your breathing can be regulated. When the breathing is regulated, your mind is able to reach a higher level of calmness. This calmness can again help you to regulate the breathing, until your mind is deep. After you have trained for a long time, your breathing will be full and slender, and your mind will be very clear. It is said: "Xin Xi Xiang Yi" (心息相依), which means "Heart (Mind) and breathing (are) mutually dependent." When you reach this meditative state, your heartbeat slows down, and your mind is very clear: you have entered the sphere of real meditation.

An ancient Daoist named Li Ching-Yen said: "Regulating breathing means to regulate the real breathing until (you) stop."[18] This means that **correct regulating means regulating is no longer necessary. Real regulating is no longer a conscious process, but has become so natural that it can be accomplished without conscious effort**. In other words, although you start by consciously regulating your breath, you must get to the point where the regulating happens naturally, and you no longer have to think about it. When you breathe, if you concentrate your mind on your breathing, then it is not true regulating, because the Qi in your lungs will become stagnant. When you reach the level of true regulating, you don't have to pay attention to it, and you can use your mind efficiently to lead the Qi. Remember, **wherev-

er the Yi is, there is the Qi. If the Yi stops in one spot, the Qi will be stagnant. It is the Yi which leads the Qi and makes it move. Therefore, when you are in a state of correct breath regulation, your mind is free. There is no sound stagnation, urgency, or hesitation, and you can finally be calm and peaceful.

You can see that when the breath is regulated correctly, the Qi will also be regulated. They are mutually related and cannot be separated. This idea is explained frequently in the Daoist literature. The Daoist Goang Cheng Zi said: "One exhale, the Earth Qi rises; one inhale, the Heaven Qi descends; real man's (meaning one who has attained the real Dao) repeated breathing at the navel, then my real Qi is naturally connected."[19] This says that when you breathe you should move your abdomen, as if you were breathing from your navel. The earth Qi is the negative (Yin) energy from your kidneys, and the sky Qi is the positive (Yang) energy which comes from the food you eat and the air you breathe. When you breathe from the navel, these two Qi's will connect and combine. Some people think that they know what Qi is, but they really don't. Once you connect the two Qi's, you will know what the "real" Qi is, and you may become a "real" man, which means to attain the Dao.

The Daoist book *Chain Dao Zhen Yen (Sing (of the) Dao (with) Real Words)* says: "One exhale one inhale to communicate Qi's function, one movement one calmness is the same as (i.e., is the source of) creation and variation."[20] The first part of this statement again implies that the functioning of Qi is connected with the breathing. The second part of this sentence means that all creation and variation come from the interaction of movement (Yang) and calmness (Yin). *Huang Ting Ching (Yellow Yard Classic)* says: "Breathe Original Qi to seek immortality."[21] In China, the traditional Daoists wore yellow robes, and they meditated in a "yard" or hall. This sentence means that in order to reach the goal of immortality, you must seek to find and understand the Original Qi which comes from the Dan Tian through correct breathing.

Moreover, the Daoist Wu Zhen Ren said: "Use the Post-Birth breathing to look for the real person's (i.e. the immortal's) breathing place."[22] In this sentence it is clear that in order to locate the immortal breathing place (the Dan Tian), you must rely on and know how to regulate your Post-Birth, or natural, breathing. Through regulating your Post-Birth breathing you will gradually be able to locate the residence of the Qi (the Dan Tian), and eventually you will be able to use your Dan Tian to breath like the immortal Daoists. Finally, in the Daoist song *Ling Yuan Da Dao Ge (The Great Daoist Song of the Spirit's Origin)* it is said: "The Originals (Original Jing, Qi, and Shen) are internally transported peacefully, so that you can become real (immortal); (if you) depend (only) on external breathing (you) will not reach the end (goal)."[23] From this song, you can see the internal breathing (breathing at the Dan Tian) is the key to training your three treasures and finally reaching immortality. However, you must first know how to regulate your external breathing correctly.

All of these emphasize the importance of breathing. There are eight key words for air breathing which a Qigong practitioner should follow during practice. Once you understand them you will be able to substantially shorten the time needed to reach your Qigong goals. These eight key words are: 1. Calm (Jing, 靜); 2. Slender (Xi, 細);

3. Deep (Shen, 深); 4. Long (Chang, 長); 5. Continuous (You, 悠); 6. Uniform (Yun, 勻);
7. Slow (Huan, 緩), and 8. Soft (Mian, 綿). These key words are self-explanatory, and
with a little thought you should be able to understand them.

Regulating the Mind (Tiao Xin, 調心)

It is said in Daoist society that: "(When) large Dao is taught, first stop thought;
when thought is not stopped, (the lessons are) in vain."[24] This means that when you
first practice Qigong, the most difficult training is to stop your thinking. The final goal
for your mind is "the thought of no thought" (無念之念). Your mind does not think of
the past, the present, or the future. Your mind is completely separated from influences of the present such as worry, happiness, and sadness. Then your mind can be
calm and steady, and can finally gain peace. Only when you are in the state of "the
thought of no thought" will you be relaxed and able to sense calmly and accurately.

Regulating your mind means using your consciousness to stop the activity in
your mind in order to set it free from the bondage of ideas, emotion, and conscious
thought. When you reach this level your mind will be calm, peaceful, empty, and
light. Then your mind has really reached the goal of relaxation. Only when you reach
this stage will you be able to relax deep into your marrow and internal organs. Only
then will your mind be clear enough to see (feel) the internal Qi circulation and to
communicate with your Qi and organs. In Daoist society it is called, "Nei Shi Gongfu"
(內視功夫), which means the Gongfu of internal vision.

When you reach this real relaxation you may be able to sense the different elements which make up your body: solid matter, liquids, gases, energy, and spirit. You
may even be able to see or feel the different colors that are associated with your five
organs—green (liver), white (lungs), black (kidneys), yellow (spleen), and red
(heart).

Once your mind is relaxed and regulated and you can sense your internal organs,
you may decide to study the five element theory. This is a very profound subject,
and it is sometimes interpreted differently by Oriental physicians and Qigong practitioners. When understood properly, it can give you a method of analyzing the interrelationships between your organs and help you devise ways to correct imbalances.

For example, the lungs correspond to the element Metal, and the heart to the element Fire. Metal (the lungs) can be used to adjust the heat of the Fire (the heart),
because metal can take a large quantity of heat away from fire, (and thus cool down
the heart). When you feel uneasy or have heartburn (excess fire in the heart), you
may use deep breathing to calm down the uneasy emotions or cool off the heartburn.

Naturally, it will take a lot of practice to reach this level. In the beginning, you
should not have any ideas or intentions, because they will make it harder for your
mind to relax and empty itself of thoughts. Once you are in a state of "no thought,"
place your attention on your Dan Tian. It is said "Yi Shou Dan Tian" (意守丹田), which
means "The Mind is kept on the Dan Tian." The Dan Tian is the origin and residence
of your Qi. Your mind can build up the Qi here (start the fire, Qi Huo, 起火), then lead
the Qi anywhere you wish, and finally lead the Qi back to its residence. When your
mind is on the Dan Tian, your Qi will always have a root. When you keep this root,

your Qi will be strong and full, and it will go where you want it to go. You can see that when you practice Qigong, your mind cannot be completely empty and relaxed. You must find the firmness within the relaxation, then you can reach your goal.

In Qigong training, it is said: "Use your Yi (Mind) to **lead** your Qi" (Yi Yi Yin Qi)(以意引氣). Notice the word **lead**. Qi behaves like water—it cannot be pushed, but it can be led. When Qi is led, it will flow smoothly and without stagnation. When it is pushed, it will flood and enter the wrong paths. Remember, wherever your Yi goes first, the Qi will naturally follow. For example, if you intend to lift an object, this intention is your Yi. This Yi will lead the Qi to the arms to energize the physical muscles, and then the object can be lifted.

It is said: "Your Yi cannot be on your Qi. Once your Yi is on your Qi, the Qi is stagnant."[25] When you want to walk from one spot to another, you must first mobilize your intention and direct it to the goal, then your body will follow. The mind must always be ahead of the body. If your mind stays on your body, you will not be able to move.

In Qigong training, the first thing is to know what Qi is. If you do not know what Qi is, how will you be able to lead it? Once you know what Qi is and experience it, then your Yi will have something to lead. The next thing in Qigong training is knowing how your Yi communicates with your Qi. That means that your Yi should be able to sense and feel the Qi flow and understand how strong and smooth it is. In Taiji Qigong society, it is commonly said that your Yi must "listen" to your Qi and "understand" it. Listen means to pay careful attention to what you sense and feel. The more you pay attention, the better you will be able to understand. Only after you understand the Qi situation will your Yi be able to set up the strategy. In Qigong your mind or Yi must generate the idea (visualize your intention), which is like an order to your Qi to complete a certain mission.

The more your Yi communicates with your Qi, the more efficiently the Qi can be led. For this reason, as a Qigong beginner you must first learn about Yi and Qi, and also learn how to help them communicate efficiently. Yi is the key in Qigong practice. Without this Yi you would not be able to lead your Qi, let alone build up the strength of the Qi or circulate it throughout your entire body.

Remember **when the Yi is strong, the Qi is strong, and when the Yi is weak, the Qi is weak**. Therefore, the first step of Qigong training is to develop your Yi. The first secret of a strong Yi is **calmness**. When you are calm, you can see things clearly and not be disturbed by surrounding distractions. With your mind calm, you will be able to concentrate.

Confucius said: "First you must be calm, then your mind can be steady. Once your mind is steady, then you are at peace. Only when you are at peace are you able to think and finally gain."[26] This procedure is also applied in meditation or Qigong exercise: First Calm, then Steady, Peace, Think, and finally Gain. When you practice Qigong, first you must learn to be emotionally calm. Once calm, you will be able to see what you want and firm your mind (steady). This firm and steady mind is your intention or Yi (it is how your Yi is generated). Only after you know what you really want will your mind gain peace and be able to relax emotionally and physically. Once you have reached this step, you must then concentrate or think in order to execute your intention. Under this thoughtful and concentrated mind, your Qi will follow and you will be able to gain what you wish.

However, the most difficult part of regulating the mind is learning how to neutralize the thoughts which keep coming back to bother you. This is especially true in still meditation practice. In still meditation, once you have entered a deep, profound meditative state, new thoughts, fantasies, your imagination, or any guilt from what you have done in the past that is hidden behind your mask will emerge and bother you. Normally, the first step of the regulating process is to stop new fantasies and images. Then, you must deal with your conscious mind. That means you must learn how to remove the mask from your face. Only then will you see yourself clearly. Therefore, the first step is to know yourself. Next, you must learn how to handle the problem instead of continuing to avoid it.

There are many ways of regulating your mind. However, the most important key to success is to use your wisdom mind to analyze the situation and find the solution. Do not let your emotional mind govern your thinking. Here, I would like to share with you a few stories about regulating the mind. Hopefully these stories can provide you with a guideline for your own regulation.

In China many centuries ago, two monks were walking side by side down a muddy road when they came upon a large puddle which completely blocked the road. A very beautiful lady in a lovely gown stood at the edge of the puddle, unable to go further without spoiling her clothes.

Without hesitation, one of the monks picked her up and carried her across the puddle, set her down on the other side, and continued on his way. Many hours later when the two monks were preparing to camp for the night, the second monk turned to the first and said, "I can no longer hold this back, I'm quite angry at you! We are not supposed to look at women, particularly pretty ones, never mind touch them. Why did you do that?" The first monk replied, "Brother, I left the woman at the mud puddle; why are you still carrying her?"

From this story, you can see that often, the thought which bothers you is created by nobody but yourself. If you can use your wisdom mind to govern yourself, many times you can set your mind free from emotional bondage regardless of the situation.

It is true that frequently the mind bothers or enslaves you to the desire for material enjoyment or money. From this desire, you misunderstand the meaning of life. **A really happy life comes from satisfaction of both material and spiritual needs**.

Have you ever thought about what the real meaning of your life is? What is the real goal for your life? Are you enslaved by money, power or love? What will make you truly happy?

I remember a story one of my professors at Taiwan University told me: "There was a jail with a prisoner in it," he said, "who was surrounded by mountains of money. He kept counting the money and feeling so happy about his life, thinking that he was the richest man in the whole world. A man passing by saw him and said through the tiny window: 'Why are you so happy? You are in prison. Do you know that?' The prisoner laughed: 'No! No! It is not that I am inside the jail, it is that you are outside of the jail!'"

How do you feel about this story? Do you want to be a prisoner and a slave to money, or do you want to be the real you and feel free internally? Think and be happy.

There is another story which was told to me by one of my students. Since I heard this story, it has always offered me a new guideline for my life. This new guideline is to appreciate what you have; only then will you have a peaceful mind. This does not mean you should not be aggressive in pursuing a better life. Keep pursuing by creating a new target and a new path for your life. It is Yang. However, often you will be depressed and discouraged from obstacles on this path. Therefore, you must also learn how to comfort yourself and appreciate what you already have. This is Yin. Only if you have both Yin and Yang can your life be happy and meaningful.

Long ago, there was a servant who served a bad tempered and impatient master. It did not matter how he tried, he was always blamed and beaten by this master. However, it was the strange truth that the servant was always happy, and his master was always sad and depressed.

One day, there was a kind man who could not understand this phenomena, and finally decided to ask this servant why he was always happy even though he was treated so badly. The servant replied: "Everyone has one day of life each day; half of the day is spent awake and the other half is spent sleeping. Although in the daytime, I am a servant and my master treats me badly, in the nighttime, I always dream that I am a king and there are thousands of servants serving me luxuriously. Look at my master: In the daytime, he is mad, depressed, greedy, and unhappy. In the nighttime, he has nightmares and cannot even have one night of nice rest. I really feel sorry for my master. Comparing me to him, I am surely happier than he is."

Friends, what do you think about this story? You are the only one responsible for your happiness. If you are not satisfied, and always complain about what you have obtained, you will be on the course of forever-unhappiness. It is said in the Western society: "If you smile, the whole world smiles with you, but if you cry, you cry alone." What an accurate saying!

Regulating the Qi (Tiao Qi, 調氣)

Before you can regulate your Qi you must first regulate your body, breath, and mind. If you compare your body to a battlefield, then your mind is like the general who generates ideas and controls the situation, and your breathing is the strategy. Your Qi is like the soldiers who are led to the most advantageous places on the battlefield. All four elements are necessary and all four must be coordinated with each other if you are to win the war against sickness and aging.

If you want to arrange your soldiers most effectively for battle, you must know which area of the battlefield is most important, and where you are weakest (where your Qi is deficient) and need to send reinforcements. If you have more soldiers than you need in one area (excessive Qi), then you can send them somewhere else where the ranks are thin. As a general, you must also know how many soldiers are available for the battle, and how many you will need for protecting yourself and your headquarters. To be successful, not only do you need good strategy (breathing), but you also need to communicate and understand the situation effectively with your troops, or all of your strategy will be in vain. When your Yi (the general) knows how to regulate the body (knows the battlefield), how to regulate breathing (set up the strategy), and how to effectively regulate Qi (direct your soldiers), you will be able to reach the final goal of Qigong training.

In order to regulate your Qi so that it moves smoothly in the correct paths, you need more than just efficient Yi-Qi communication. You also need to know how to generate Qi. If you do not have enough Qi in your body, how can you regulate it? In a battle, if you do not have enough soldiers to set up your strategy, you have already lost.

When you practice Qigong, you must first train to make your Qi flow naturally and smoothly. There are some Qigong exercises in which you intentionally hold your Yi, and thus hold your Qi, in a specific area. As a beginner, however, you should first learn how to make the Qi flow smoothly instead of building a Qi dam, which is commonly done in external martial Qigong training.

In order to make the Qi flow naturally and smoothly, your Yi must first be relaxed. Only when your Yi is relaxed will your body be relaxed and the Qi channels open for the Qi to circulate. Then you must coordinate your Qi flow with your breathing. Breathing regularly and calmly will make your Yi calm, and allow your body to relax even more.

Regulating the Spirit (Tiao Shen, 調神)

There is one thing that is more important than anything else in a battle, and that is fighting spirit. You may have the best general, who knows the battlefield well and is also an expert strategist, but if his soldiers do not have a high fighting spirit (morale), he might still lose. Remember, **spirit is the center and root of a fight**. When you keep this center, one soldier can be equal to ten soldiers. When his spirit is high, a soldier will obey his orders accurately and willingly, and his general will be able to control the situation efficiently. In a battle, in order for a soldier to have this kind of morale, he must know why he is fighting, how to fight, and what he can expect after the fight. Under these conditions, he will know what he is doing and why, and this understanding will raise his spirit, strengthen his will, and increase his patience and endurance.

Shen, which is the Chinese term for spirit, originates from the Yi (the general). When the Shen is strong, the Yi is firm. When the Yi is firm, the Shen will be steady and calm. **The Shen is the mental part of a soldier. When the Shen is high, the Qi is strong and easily directed. When the Qi is strong, the Shen is also strong**.

To the religious Qigong practitioners, the goal of regulating the spirit is to set the spirit free from the bondage of the physical body, and thus reach the stage of Buddhahood or enlightenment. To layman practitioners, the goal of regulating the spirit is to keep the spirit of living high to prevent the body from getting sick and degenerating. It is often seen that, before a person retires, he has good health. However, once retired, he will get sick easily and his physical condition will deteriorate quickly. When you are working, your spirit remains high and alert. This keeps the Qi circulating smoothly in the body.

All of these training concepts and procedures are common to all Chinese Qigong. To reach a deep level of understanding and penetrate to the essence of any Qigong practice, you should always keep these five training criteria in mind and examine them for deeper levels of meaning. This is the only way to gain the real mental and physical health benefits from your training. Always remember that Qigong training is not just the forms. Your feelings and comprehension are the essential roots of the entire training. This Yin side of the training has no limit, and the deeper you understand, the better you will see how much more there is to know.

1-6. How to Use This Book

When you practice any Qigong, you must first ask: What, Why, and How. "What" means: "What am I looking for?" "What do I expect?" and "What should I do?" Then you must ask: "Why do I need it?" "Why does it work?" "Why must I do it this way instead of that way?" Finally, you must determine: "How does it work?" "How much have I advanced toward my goal?" And "How will I be able to advance further?"

It is very important to understand what you are practicing, not just automatically to repeat what you have learned. Understanding is the root of any work. With understanding you will be able to know your goal. Once you know your goal, your mind can be firm and steady. With this understanding, you will be able to see why something has happened, and what the principles and theories behind it are. Without all of this, your work will be done blindly, and it will be a long and painful process. Only when you are sure what your target is and why you need to reach it should you raise the question of how you are going to accomplish it. The answers to all of these questions form the root of your practice, and will help you to avoid the wondering and confusion that uncertainty brings. If you keep this root, you will be able to apply the theory and make it grow—you will know how to create. Without this root, what you learn will be only branches and flowers, and in time they will wither.

In China there is a story about an old man who was able to change a piece of rock into gold. One day, a boy came to see him and asked for his help. The old man said: "Boy! What do you want? Gold? I can give you all of the gold you want." The boy replied: "No, Master, what I want is not your gold. What I want is the trick of how to change the rock into gold!" When you just have gold, you can spend it all and become poor again. If you have the trick of how to make gold, you will never be poor. For the same reason, when you learn Qigong you should learn the theory and principle behind it, not just the practice. Understanding theory and principle will not only shorten your time of pondering and practice, but also enable you to practice most efficiently.

This book has a companion videotape, *Back Pain,* also available from YMAA Publication Center. One of the hardest parts of the training process is learning how actually to do the forms correctly. Every Qigong movement has its special meaning and purpose. In order to make sure your movements or forms are correct, it is best to work with the tape and book together. There are some important aspects which you may not be able to pick up from reading, but once you see them, they will be clear. There are other important ideas for which it was impossible to take the time to explain in the videotape, such as the theory and principles; these can only be explained in the book. It cannot be denied that under the tutelage of a master you can learn more quickly and perfectly than is possible using only tapes and books. What you are missing is the master's experience and feeling. However, if you ponder carefully and practice patiently and perseveringly, you will be able to make up for this lack through your own experience and practice. This book and the tape are designed for self-instruction. You will find that they will serve you as a key to enter into the field of Qigong.

References

1. "Backaches," Oliver Fultz, *American Health,* November 1991.

2. "Outpatient Management of Low Back Pain," Judith A. Chase, *Orthopedic Nursing*, January/February 1992, Vol 11/No. 1.

3. "Life's Invisible Current," by Albert L. Huebner, *East West Journal,* June 1986.

4. *The Body Electric*, by Robert O. Becker, M.D. and Gary Selden, Quill, William Morrow, New York, 1985.

5. *"Healing with Nature's Energy,"* by Richard Leviton, *East West Journal,* June 1986.

6. *A Child is Born*, by Lennart Nilsson, A DTP/Seymour Lawrence Book, 1990.

7. 解剖生理學 (*A Study of Anatomic Physiology*)
   李文森編著。華杏出版股份有限公司。Taipei, 1986.

8. *Grant's Atlas of Anatomy*, James E. Anderson, 7th Edition, Williams & Wilkins Co., 9-92, 1978.

9. "Complex and Hidden Brain in the Gut Makes Stomachaches and Butterflies," Sandra Blakeslee, *The New York Times,* January 23, 1996.

10. *Bioenergetics*, by Albert L. Lehninger, pp. 5-6, W. A, Benjamin, Inc. Menlo Park, California, 1971.

11. *Photographic Anatomy of the Human Body*, by J. W. Rohen, 邯鄲出版社，Taipei, Taiwan, 1984.

12. "Restoring Ebbing Hormones May Slow Aging," by Jane E. Brody, *The New York Times,* July 18, 1995.

13. 莊子曰：〝眞人之息以踵，眾人之息以喉。〞

14. 人生七十古來稀。

15. 一百二十謂之天。

16. Before birth, you have no Qi of your own, but rather you use your mother's Qi. When you are born, you start creating Qi from the Original Essence (Yuan Jing) which you received from your parents. This Qi is called Pre-Birth Qi, as well as Original Qi. It is also called Pre-Heaven Qi (Xian Tian Qi) because it comes from the Original Jing which you received before you saw the heavens (which here means the sky), i.e., before your birth.

17. 形不正，則氣不順。氣不順，則意不寧。意不寧，則氣散亂。

18. 調息要調無息息。

19. 廣成子曰：一呼則地氣上升，一吸則天氣下降，人之反覆呼吸於蒂，則我之眞氣自然相接。

20. 唱道眞言曰：一呼一吸通乎氣機，一動一靜同乎造化。

21. 黃庭經曰：呼吸元氣以求仙。

22. 伍眞人曰：用後天之呼吸，尋眞人呼吸處。

23. 靈源大道歌曰：元和內運即成眞，呼吸外求終未了。

24. 大道教人先止念，念頭不住亦徒然

25. 意不在氣，在氣則滯。

26. 孔子曰：先靜爾后有定，定爾后能安，安爾后能慮，慮爾后能得。

CHAPTER 2

Understanding Our Back

背的構造

2-1. Introduction

In order to maintain the health of our back, or solve back pain problems, the first step is to study the anatomical structure of our back—especially the spine. From this study, we can better understand the problem and its possible causes. In addition, according to Chinese medical science, many back pain problems may also be caused from Qi imbalance or stagnation in the spine or back muscles. Therefore, if we are wise, we should examine our back from both a Western physical understanding and also from an Eastern comprehension of the Qi distribution in our back.

In the next section of this chapter, we will summarize the physical anatomical structure of our back. Then, in section 2-3, we will review the Qi distribution network from a Chinese medical point of view. This synthesis of Western physical science and Eastern bioenergetic science will provide a more complete paradigm from which to analyze the factors that can affect your lower back.

2-2. Anatomical Structure of Our Back

Underneath the skin of our back, there are many sets of muscles. These muscles allow us to move our body. We can also see many nerve endings emerging from the muscles and spreading from the center to the sides (Figure 2-1). Beneath the muscles are the spine and the ribs (Figure 2-2). Most importantly, the peripheral nervous system (PNS) branches out from the spinal cord (Figure 2-3). The nerves branch out from the spinal cord to the arms through the cervical (C5-C8) and thoracic (T1) vertebrae, whereas the nerves from the lower portion of the spinal cord extend to the hips and legs through the lumbar vertebrae (L2-L5) and sacrum (S1-S5)(Figures 2-4 and 2-5). In addition, almost all of the nerves branching out from the spinal cord

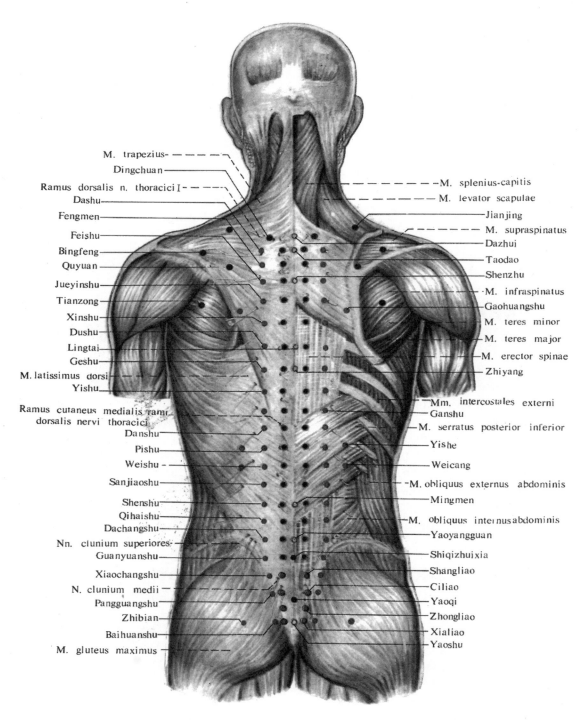

Figure 2-1. Superficial Anatomical Structure of the Posterior Aspect of the Trunk

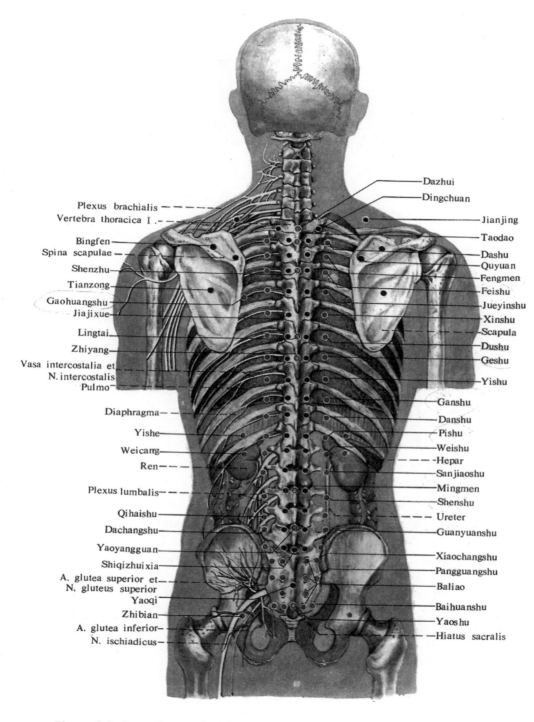

Figure 2-2. Deep Anatomical Structure of the Posterior Aspect of the Trunk

Dazhui
Dingchuan
Jianjing
Taodao
Dashu
Quyuan
Fengmen
Feishu
Jueyinshu
Xinshu
Scapula
Dushu
Geshu
Yishu
Ganshu
Danshu
Pishu
Weishu
Hepar
Sanjiaoshu
Mingmen
Shenshu
Ureter
Guanyuanshu
Xiaochangshu
Pangguangshu
Baliao
Baihuanshu
Yaoshu
Hiatus sacralis

Plexus brachialis
Vertebra thoracica I
Bingfen
Spina scapulae
Shenzhu
Tianzong
Gaohuangshu
Jiajixue
Lingtai
Zhiyang
Vasa intercostalia et
N. intercostalis
Pulmo
Diaphragma
Yishe
Weicang
Ren
Plexus lumbalis
Qihaishu
Dachangshu
Yaoyangguan
Shiqizhuixia
A. glutea superior et
N. gluteus superior
Yaoqi
Zhibian
A. glutea inferior
N. ischiadicus

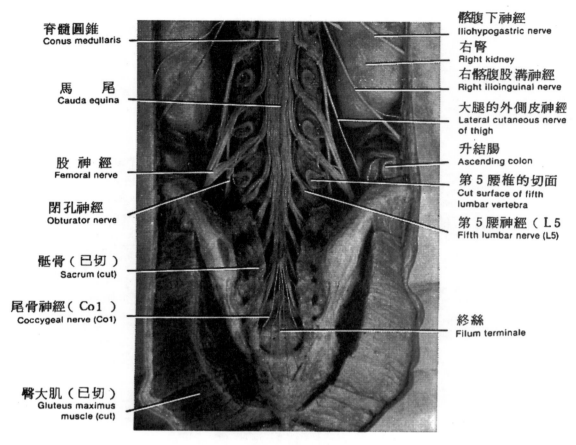

脊髓圆錐
Conus medullaris

馬　尾
Cauda equina

股　神　經
Femoral nerve

閉孔神經
Obturator nerve

骶骨（已切）
Sacrum (cut)

尾骨神經（ Co1 ）
Coccygeal nerve (Co1)

臀大肌（已切）
Gluteus maximus
muscle (cut)

髂腹下神經
Iliohypogastric nerve

右腎
Right kidney

右髂腹股 溝神經
Right ilioinguinal nerve

大腿的外側皮神經
Lateral cutaneous nerve
of thigh

升結腸
Ascending colon

第 5 腰椎的切面
Cut surface of fifth
lumbar vertebra

第 5 腰神經（ L 5 ）
Fifth lumbar nerve (L5)

終絲
Filum terminale

Figure 2-3. Nerves Branch Out (PNS) from the Spinal Cord (CNS)

connect to various sensory organs and viscera, especially the nerves in the area of the thoracic vertebrae (Figure 2-6). It is from these connections that our brain is able to sense our entire body and control it. Whenever there is a problem at any verte-bra, corresponding organs or areas of the body will neither send nor receive clear impulses from the brain. We perceive such a disturbance as pain. Therefore, the physical health of your spine is one of the most important and critical requirements for your health.

Next, we will discuss the general structure of the spine. We will then review the nervous system in the back. Finally, since most back problems occur in the lower back, we will briefly summarize the structure of the lower back area.

About the Spine[1 & 2]

The spine is an extremely complex and elegant structure, made up of **vertebrae**, **discs**, the **spinal cord**, and **nerves**. Although we are born with 33 separate vertebrae, by adulthood most of us have only 24. The nine vertebrae at the base of the spine

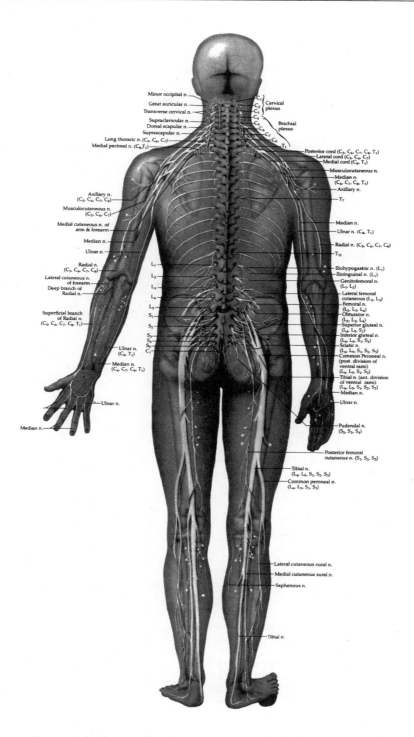

Figure 2-4. Nerves Distribution from the Spinal Cord to the Limbs
(© Anatomical Chart Co., Skokie, IL.)

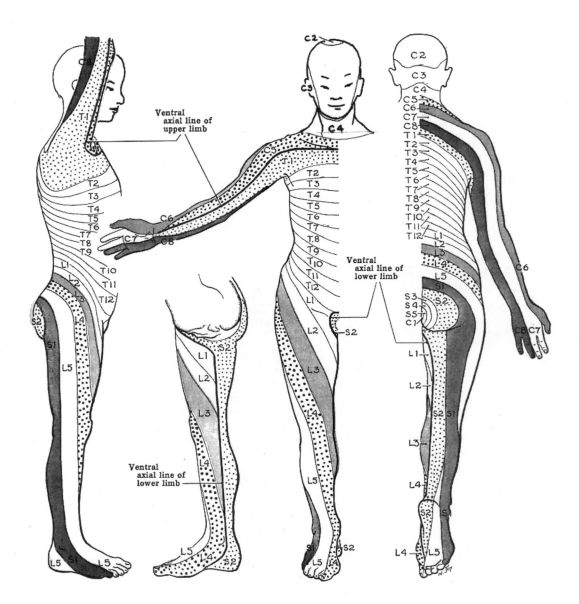

Figure 2-5. Dermatomes of the Upper and Lower Limbs

grow together. The upper five form a triangular bone and become the **sacrum**. The lowest four form the tailbone or coccyx, and often fuse with the sacrum above (Figure 2-7).

Physicians use a code to identify the vertebrae. The seven in the neck—the cervical vertebrae that support and provide movement for the head—are called C1 to C7. The thoracic vertebrae, numbered T1 to T12, join with and are supported by the

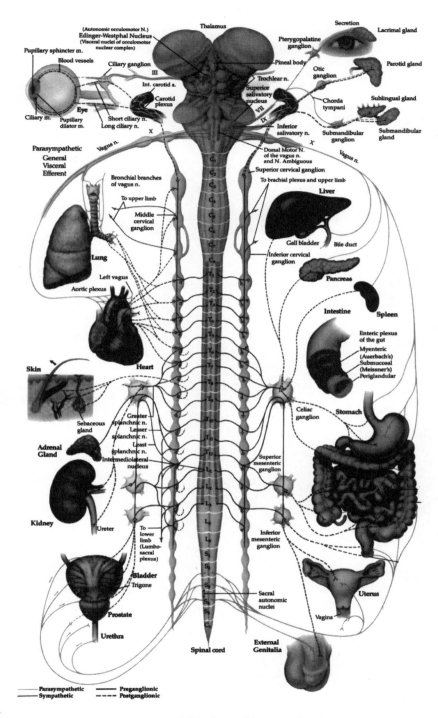

**Figure 2-6. A Schematic Representation of the Autonomic
Nervous System and the Organs it Serves**
(© Anatomical Chart Co., Skokie, IL.)

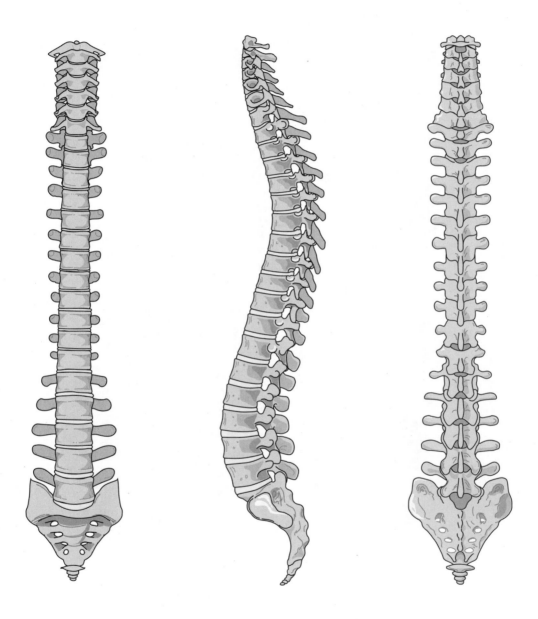

Figure 2-7. Anterior View, Left Lateral View, and Posterior View of the Spinal Column

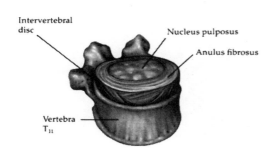

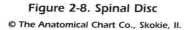

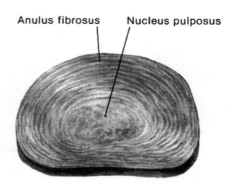

Figure 2-8. Spinal Disc
© The Anatomical Chart Co., Skokie, Il.

Figure 2-9. Structure of Intervertebral Disc
(Frank H. Netter, M.D. The Ciba Collection of Medical
Illustrations, vol. 1, The Nervous System, © 1983 Novartis)

ribs, which protect the heart and lungs. Because they are fairly rigid, thoracic vertebrae don't permit much movement, and consequently are not injured as often as the other vertebrae. The lumbar vertebrae, numbered L1 to L5, are located below the thoracic vertebrae and above the sacrum. These are most frequently involved in back pain, mainly because they carry most of the body's weight and stress.

The vertebrae are not stacked one on top of the other in a straight line. Rather, each rests on the one below at an angle, forming an S-curve when viewed from the side. The vertebrae would collapse without the tough ligaments that secure them together, and the strong muscles and tendons that keep the spinal column upright.

Sandwiched between each pair of adjacent vertebrae is a spinal disc, 23 in all (Figure 2-8). Discs are flat, round structures (about one-quarter to three-quarters of an inch thick) composed of tough, fibrous outer rings of tissue that contain a soft, white jelly-like center (Figure 2-9). They actually grow larger at night. While we are resting they absorb fluid from surrounding tissues. During the day, when we are active, the weight of the spine causes some of this fluid to ooze out, making us all a little bit shorter at the end of the day.

Each disc is connected to the vertebrae above and below it by flat circular plates of cartilage. These flexible, flat pads not only keep the vertebra apart, but act as cushions between the hard bones. They compress when weight is put on them and spring back when the weight is removed (Figure 2-10). Just like a car's shock absorbers, discs can degenerate from excessive stress or from just the wear and tear of daily life. But unlike a car's shocks, the cushiony discs cannot be replaced in kind. Sometimes a bone graft can be inserted in place of a damaged disc, but so far science and medicine have found no replacement that can absorb the body's shocks.

While we need the strong, solid parts of the lumbar vertebrae to bear the body's weight, only joints will allow us to bend forward and backward, or to twist and turn. These joints are found in a ring-like structure of bone, known as the arch, located at

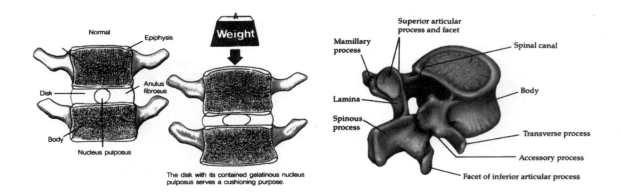

Figure 2-10. Function of Intervertebral Disc
(© Anatomical Chart Co., Skokie, IL.)

Figure 2-11. Structure of the Spinal Joint (Second Lumbar Vertebra)
(© Anatomical Chart Co., Skokie, IL.)

the rear of each vertebra. The arch has a hollow center and little bones that go off in several directions, serving as anchors for muscles and ligaments (Figure 2-11). A pair of vertical bones projecting upward and another pair projecting downward—the facet joints—glide on similar smooth-surfaced bones in the vertebrae above and below them, creating an interlocking column of bones (Figure 2-12). The hollow areas of the arches form a channel (spinal canal) that encloses and protects the spinal cord. The only parts of the spine that we can feel with our fingers are projections from the bony rings called spinous (thorn-like) processes. Each spinous process bends down slightly over the one below it to form an extra shield for the spinal cord.

The spinal cord, an extension of the brain, extends as far down as L1, where it ends in a sheaf of nerves (cauda equina) resembling a horse's tail (Figure 2-13). Throughout the length of the spine, 31 pairs of nerves branch off from the spinal cord to serve all parts of the body, transmitting sensory message of the brain (e.g., the water is cold) and messages from the brain to the muscles (e.g., lift your arm)(Figure 2-14). Where the nerves exit from the spinal cord through spaces (foramina) between adjacent vertebrae, they are called nerve roots. Few people are aware that if the neck is bent forward as far as it will go, the whole spinal cord moves upward in the spinal canal. Anything that prevents the cord and nerves from moving freely, such as abnormal bone growth within the spinal canal, will cause tingling or pain.

Thirty-three vertebrae, 23 discs, 31 pairs of spinal nerves, 140 muscles that hook on to the vertebrae, plus ligaments, tendons, cartilage—all very complicated and all potential sources of back trouble. Small wonder that in 80 percent of the cases doctors cannot pinpoint the cause of back pain. Next, let us look at the nervous system in our back.

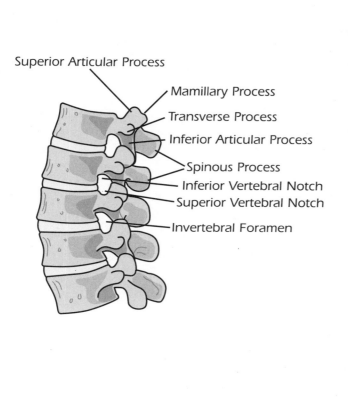

Superior Articular Process

Mamillary Process

Transverse Process

Inferior Articular Process

Spinous Process

Inferior Vertebral Notch

Superior Vertebral Notch

Invertebral Foramen

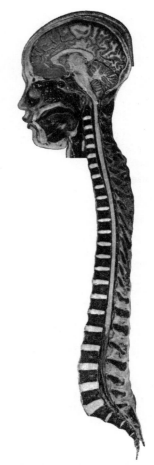

**Figure 2-12. Connecting Structure
of the Vertebrae**

**Figure 2-13. Spinal Cord Extending
From the Brain to Tailbone**

The Nervous System in the Back

A nerve is a bundle of fibers joining the central nervous system to the organs and other parts of the body. Nerves relay sensory stimuli as well as motor impulses from different parts of the body to one another.

All multicellular animals except sponges possess nervous systems. They are essentially regulatory mechanisms, controlling internal bodily functions and responses to external stimuli. The human nervous system is made up of two component sub-systems: the central nervous system (CNS) and the peripheral nervous system (PNS)(Figure 2-15).

Making up the central nervous system (CNS) are the brain and the spinal cord, which are contained and protected within the skull and the spine respectively. The CNS integrates, interprets, and transmits messages to and from the brain and the periphery of the body.

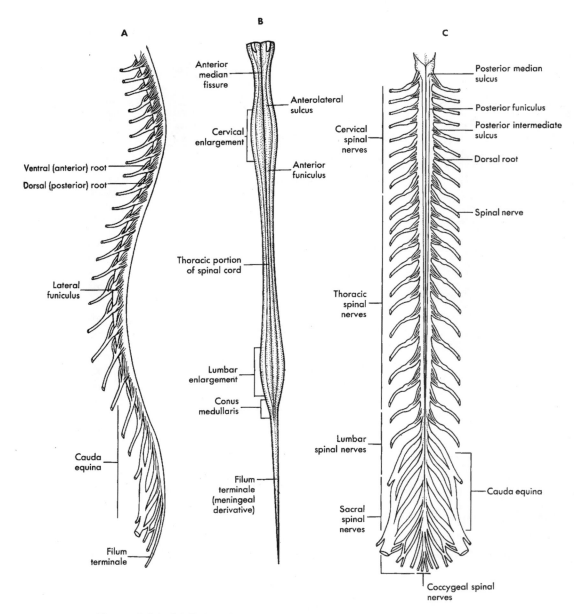

Figure 2-14. 31 Pairs of Nerves Branch Off from the Spinal Cord
J. Robert McClintic, Human Anatomy, St. Louis, 1983, Mosby-Year Book, Inc.)

Making up the peripheral nervous system (PNS) is all the nerve tissue found outside of the skull and spinal column, including not only the nerve fibers that carry impulses, but also groupings of fibers (plexuses) and nerve cell bodies (ganglions) that are found in the periphery. The PNS registers changes in internal and external environments of the body, transmitting this information to the CNS for action, and then delivering the orders of the CNS to muscles and glands for response.

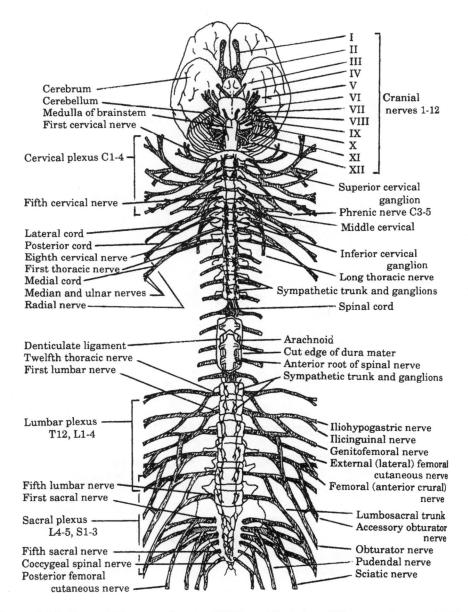

Cerebrum
Cerebellum
Medulla of brainstem
First cervical nerve

I
II
III
IV
V
VI
VII
VIII
IX
X
XI
XII

Cranial nerves 1-12

Cervical plexus C1-4

Fifth cervical nerve

Lateral cord
Posterior cord
Eighth cervical nerve
First thoracic nerve
Medial cord
Median and ulnar nerves
Radial nerve

Superior cervical ganglion
Phrenic nerve C3-5
Middle cervical
Inferior cervical ganglion
Long thoracic nerve
Sympathetic trunk and ganglions
Spinal cord

Denticulate ligament
Twelfth thoracic nerve
First lumbar nerve

Arachnoid
Cut edge of dura mater
Anterior root of spinal nerve
Sympathetic trunk and ganglions

Lumbar plexus
T12, L1-4

Iliohypogastric nerve
Ilicinguinal nerve
Genitofemoral nerve
External (lateral) femoral cutaneous nerve
Femoral (anterior crural) nerve

Fifth lumbar nerve
First sacral nerve

Sacral plexus
L4-5, S1-3

Lumbosacral trunk
Accessory obturator nerve

Fifth sacral nerve
Coccygeal spinal nerve
Posterior femoral cutaneous nerve

Obturator nerve
Pudendal nerve
Sciatic nerve

Figure 2-15. Central Nervous System (CNS) and Peripheral Nervous System (PNS)

The PNS includes 12 pairs of cranial nerves which attach to the brain and their associated ganglions, as well as 31 pairs of spinal nerves and their ganglions. Finally, the PNS also includes specialized receptors and endings on muscles.

In terms of the function and interaction of all these constituent components, the PNS is simple yet efficient. It is "built" out of somatic fibers (somatic nervous system) that provide the nerves for the skeletal muscles as well as the skin's special

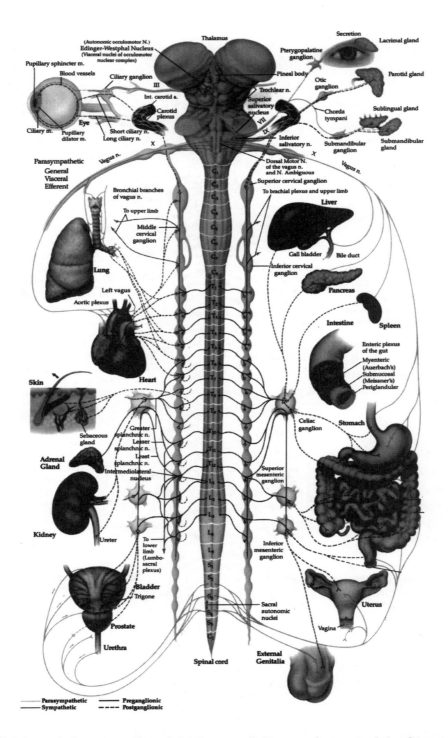

Figure 2-16. A Schematic Representation of the Autonomic Nervous System and the Organs It Serves.
(© Anatomical Chart Co., Skokie, IL.)

receptors (for touch, pressure, heat, cold), and autonomic fibers (autonomic nervous system). The autonomic fibers carry impulses to cardiac muscles and glands, and from visceral receptors (Figure 2-16). These fibers make possible the reflexes which control breathing, heart rate, blood pressure and other bodily functions in an involuntary and unbroken manner. Most organs receive fibers from two subdivisions of the autonomic nervous system. The parasympathetic (craniosacral) division is comprised of certain cranial nerves and several of the sacral spinal nerves, and furnishes nervous influences for the purpose of conservation of body sources and maintenance of nominal function levels. The sympathetic (thoracolumbar) division is comprised of the thoracic and lumber spinal nerves, and furnishes impulses for the purpose of elevating body activity in order to tolerate or resist stressful or hazardous situations. In this way an organ may have its operation intensified or diminished according to the demands of a survival situation.

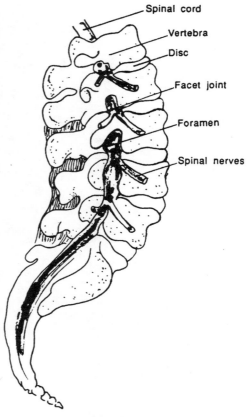

Figure 2-17. Anatomy of the Lumbar Spine

This brief anatomical discussion of the nervous system shows us that the brain and spinal cord are the center of our feeling and functioning. We have seen that nerves from the spinal cord extend out and connect to the entire body, including the limbs and also the internal organs.

There are a number of other facts about the nervous system that are also important. First, our state of mind is linked to the condition of our physical body through our nervous system. This means that if we are mentally tense or relaxed, our physical body will react accordingly. Second, the nervous system is constructed of fibrous tissues, which are part of the material side of our body. In order to function properly, or even to stay alive, this material needs Qi (bioelectricity). Third, if we compare the system of Qi distribution with the nervous system, we see that although they are related, they are not the same system. The Qi circulatory system does not supply Qi only to the nervous system, it supplies it to all of the body's cells.

The nervous system plays a critical role in the practice of Qigong healing for lower back pain. The nervous system enables us to feel what is going on everywhere in our body. Since the mind leads the Qi, if we want to lead Qi somewhere, we have to be able to feel that place. If we cannot feel that place, then the mind cannot lead the Qi there, since it has no reference to act as a guide.

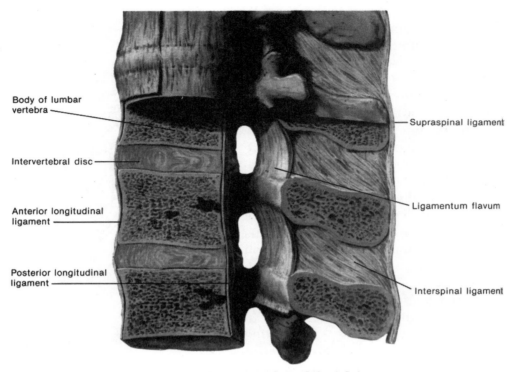

Body of lumbar vertebra

Intervertebral disc

Anterior longitudinal ligament

Posterior longitudinal ligament

Supraspinal ligament

Ligamentum flavum

Interspinal ligament

Figure 2-18. Ligaments of the Spinal Column
(Frank H. Netter, M.D. The Ciba Collection of Medical Illustratiuons, vol. 1, The Nervous System, Plate 16, © 1983 Novartis)

The nervous system is responsible for our ability to feel, and it is our ability to feel that governs the Qi. This means that the condition of the nervous system is directly related to the Qi circulation in our body. Therefore, while in Qigong healing we should pay particular attention to the Qi system, the nervous system should be second in our priorities.

Next, since most back problems occur in the lower back, it is essential for us to understand the anatomy of the lumbar spine. The more we can understand this structure, the better we can envision the condition of our lower back and devise a way to correct any problems.

Anatomical Structure of the Lumbar Spine[3]

There are normally five lumbar vertebrae (Figure 2-17). The lumbar vertebral bodies are the largest of the vertebrae because of their weight-bearing functions. The vertebrae have both facet and inter vertebral joints. The inferior facet joint from the vertebra above and the superior facet joint from the vertebra below form the facet joint. These joints are diarthrodial with synovial linings. That means that they permit relatively free movement. The inter vertebral joints (between the vertebral bodies) are amphiarthrodial, a type of cartilaginous joint allowing little motion. These joints contain fibrocartilaginous discs consisting of avascular nucleus pulposus surrounded by annulus fibrosus. As explained earlier, the discs act as shock absorbers, dissipating mechanical stress.

The vertebrae are surrounded by five different groups of ligaments that support and strengthen the spine (Figure 2-18). The lumbar vertebrae contain the spinal nerves, which exit at each level between the vertebrae through the neural foramen. The sinu-vertebral nerve is the major sensory nerve serving the structures of the lumbar spine.

Lumbar arteries arising from the aorta supply the vertebrae and ligaments with blood. The discs have no active blood supply and receive nourishment from the transfer of tissue fluid across the end plates of the disc by mechanical means. Three muscle groups support and move the lumbar spine. The erector spinae are the prominent paraspinal muscles of the lumbar spine. These muscles, in combination with the interspinales (muscles which run parallel to the spine), extend the lumbar spine. The abdominal and iliopsoas provide bending actuation (i.e., flexion).

2-3. The Qi Network in Our Back

As explained in the last chapter, we have two bodies, the physical body and the Qi body (or bioelectric body). The physical body can be seen, but Qi can only be felt. The Qi body is the vital source of the physical body (i.e., any living cells) and the foundation of our lives. The Qi body is not only related to our cells, but also to our thinking and spirit, since it is the main energy source to maintain the brain's func-tioning. Therefore, any Qi imbalance or stagnation will be the root and cause of any physical sickness or mental disorder.

Western medical science has long been studying the physical body, and ignoring the Qi body for the most part. This has begun to change in the last two decades. Therefore, the scientific understanding of the Qi body, and how it affects our health and longevity, is still in its infancy. Under these circumstances, we may still accept the ancient Chinese understanding of our body's Qi network.

In this section, we will first briefly describe this network. Then, we will focus on the central energy system and central energy lines discovered through Chinese Qigong and its possible linkage to newer scientific discovery.

Twelve Primary Qi Channels and the Eight Vessels

From the understanding of Chinese medicine, the Qi circulatory system in a human body includes eight vessels (Ba Mai, 八脈), twelve primary Qi channels (Shi Er Jing, 十二經), and thousands of secondary channels branching out from the pri-mary channels (Luo, 絡). On two of the vessels (Governing and Conception Vessels) and the twelve primary Qi channels, there are more than seven hundred acupunc-ture cavities through which the Qi level in the channels can be adjusted and regu-lated. From this Qi adjustment, the Qi circulation in the body, especially in the inter-nal organs, can be regulated into a harmonious state, the body's sickness can be cured and health can be maintained. Here, we will briefly review these three circu-latory networks. The cavities on the back which are related to back pain healing will be discussed in chapter 6. If you are interested in learning more about this Qi net-work, you may refer to Chinese acupuncture books or the book: *The Root of Chinese Qigong*, from YMAA Publication Center.

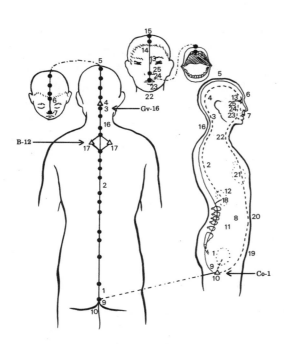

Figure 2-19. The Governing
Vessel (Du Mai)

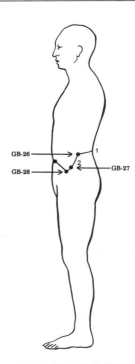

Figure 2-20. The Belt (Girdle)
Vessel (Ren Mai)

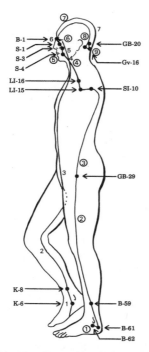

Figure 2-21. The Yang Heel Vessel (Yangchiao
Mai) and The Yin Heel Vessel (Yinchiao Mai)

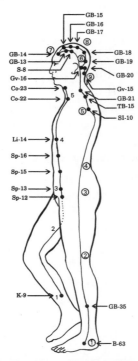

Figure 2-22. The Yang Linking Vessel (Yangwei
Mai) and The Yin Linking Vessel (Yinwei Mai)

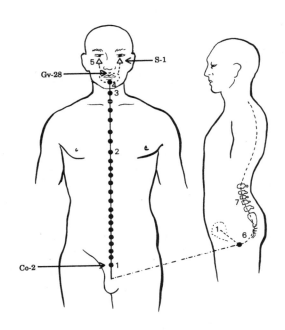

Figure 2-23. The Conception Vessel (Ren Mai)

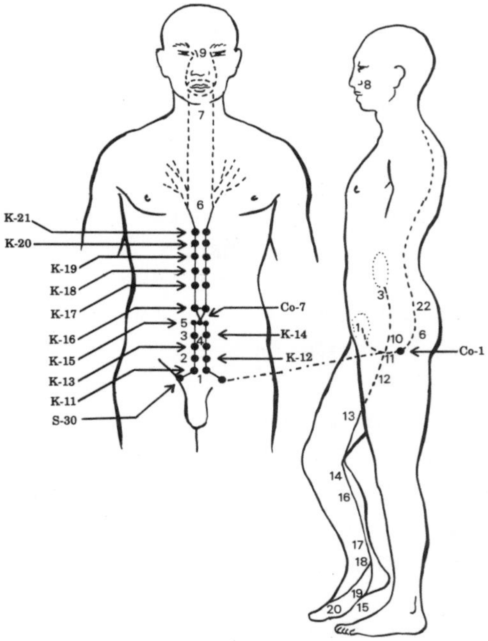

Figure 2-24. The Thrusting Vessel (Chong Mai)

Eight Vessels (Ba Mai, 八脈)

1. The Eight Vessels include four Yang vessels and four Yin vessels. They therefore balance each other.

2. **The Four Yang Vessels are:**

   Governing Vessel (Du Mai, 督脈)(Figure 2-19)

   Belt (or Girdle) Vessel (Dai Mai, 帶脈)(Figure 2-20)

   Yang Heel Vessel (Yangchiao Mai, 陽蹻脈)(Figure 2-21)

   Yang Linking Vessel (Yangwei Mai, 陽維脈)(Figure 2-22)

   The Four Yin Vessels are:

   Conception Vessel (Ren Mai, 任脈)(Figure 2-23)

   Thrusting Vessel (Chong Mai, 衝脈)(Figure 2-24)

   Yin Heel Vessel (Yinchiao Mai, 陰蹻脈)(Figure 2-21)

   Yin Linking Vessel (Yinwei Mai, 陰維脈)(Figure 2-22).

3. According to Chinese medicine, vessels function as reservoirs, connected to the twelve primary Qi channels and regulating the Qi level circulating in these channels. When the Qi level in some specific channel is too high, one or more of the reservoirs will absorb the excess Qi, and if the Qi is too low,

the shortfall will be supplied from these vessels. Consequently, a harmonious level can be maintained.

4. The two Yang vessels, Governing and Belt Vessels, and the two Yin vessels, Conception and Thrusting Vessels, are individual and are located in the torso. The other four vessels exist in pairs, and are located in the legs. There are no vessels in the arms.

5. Among the eight vessels, according to Chinese medicine, the Governing and Conception Vessels are the most important, since they are the main vessels which regulate the twelve primary Qi channels. The Governing Vessel regulates the Qi in the six primary Yang Qi channels, while the Conception Vessel regulates the Qi in the six primary Yin Qi Channels. There are acupuncture cavities on these two vessels, and none on the other six vessels. However, there are many cavities on these six vessels which belong to the twelve primary Qi channels. These cavities are considered to be gates which allow the Qi to pass between the vessels and channels.

6. According to Chinese Qigong practice for health and longevity, the methods of learning how to fill out the Qi in the vessels are very important. The reason for this is that these eight vessels are the reservoirs for the Qi. When the Qi in these reservoirs is abundant, the Qi regulating potential of the primary Qi channels will be high and efficient. Among these eight vessels, the Governing and Conception Vessels are the most important, since they regulate the twelve primary Qi channels. The Qi circulates in these two vessels and distributes to the twelve primary Qi channels (i.e., limbs) throughout the day.

7. In Religious Qigong meditation practice for enlightenment, the Thrusting Vessel (i.e., spinal cord) is very important. The Thrusting Vessel connects the brain and the perineum, and the Qi is abundant in this vessel at around midnight. Traditionally, during the midnight hours, we are sleeping and the physical body is extremely relaxed. In this situation, the physical body does not need a great amount of Qi to support its activities, and the Qi circulates abundantly in the spinal cord to nourish the brain and sexual organs. Hormone production is therefore increased at night. When the brain is nourished and its function is raised a high level, the spirit can be raised and enlightenment can be achieved. If you are interested in more on this subject, please refer to the book: *Muscle/Tendon Changing and Marrow/Brain Washing Chi Kung,* from YMAA Publication Center.

8. The Governing Vessel, which is located at the center of the back, is the main vessel supplying Qi to the nervous system branching out from the spinal cord. The nervous system is constructed of physical cells which need to be nourished with Qi (bioelectricity) to function and stay alive. This tells us that Qi is ultimately the root of the nerves' functioning. To maintain abundant Qi circulation in this vessel, your physical health condition is extremely impor-

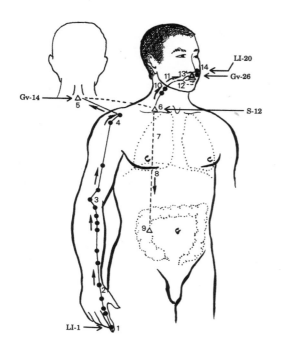

Figure 2-25. Arm Yang Brightness Large Intestine Channel

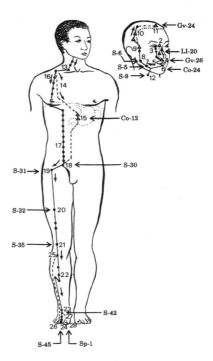

Figure 2-26. Leg Yang Brightness Stomach Channel

tant. If there is any physical injury or damage along the course of this vessel, the Qi supply to the nervous system will be stagnant and irregular. Moreover, in order to have healthy and abundant Qi circulation in this vessel, you must learn how to increase the storage of the Qi in the Lower Dan Tian, which is the main Qi reservoir or bioelectric battery in our body.

9. The Yang Belt Vessel is the only vessel in which the Qi circulates horizontally. To Qigong practitioners, this vessel is very important. Since the Qi status in this vessel is Yang, the Qi is expanding outward. It is from this vessel that we feel our balance. It is just like an airplane or a tight-rope walker, the longer the wings or the balancing pole, the easier it will be to find and maintain balance. A Qigong practitioner or a Chinese martial artist will train this vessel and make the Qi expand outward further, therefore increasing the balance and stability of both the physical and mental bodies. When you have more balance and stability, you can find your center. When you find your physical and mental center, then you will be rooted. Once you are rooted, your spirit can be raised to a higher level.

The Twelve Primary Qi Channels and Their Branches (Shi Er Jing Luo, 十二經絡)

1. The twelve primary Qi Channels include six Yang channels and six Yin channels. They therefore balance each other.

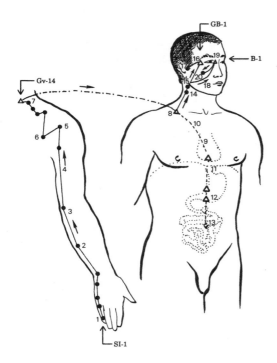

Figure 2-27. Arm Greater Yang Small Intestine Channel

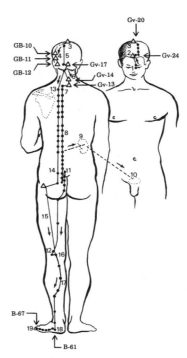

Figure 2-28. Leg Greater Yang Bladder Channel

2. **The Six Yang channels are:**

Arm Yang Brightness Large Intestine Channel (Shou Yang Ming Da Chang Jing, 手陽明大腸經)(Figure 2-25)

Leg Yang Brightness Stomach Channel (Zu Yang Ming Wei Jing, 足陽明胃經)(Figure 2-26)

Arm Greater Yang Small Intestine Channel (Shou Tai Yang Xiao Chang Jing, 手太陽小腸經)(Figure 2-27)

Leg Greater Yang Bladder Channel (Zu Tai Yang Pang Guang Jing, 足太陽膀胱經)(Figure 2-28)

Arm Lesser Yang Triple Burner Channel (Shou Shao Yang San Jiao Jing, 手少陽三焦經)(Figure 2-29)

Leg Lesser Yang Gall Bladder Channel (Zu Shao Yang Dan Jing, 足少陽膽經)(Figure 2-30)

The Six Yin channels are:

Arm Greater Yin Lung Channel (Shou Tai Yin Fei Jing, 手太陰肺經) (Figure 2-31)

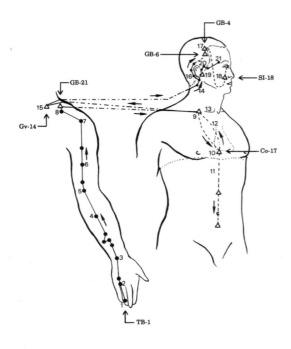

Figure 2-29. Arm Lesser Yang Triple Burner Channel

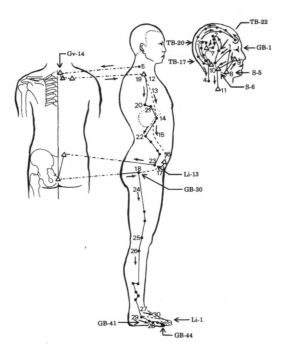

Figure 2-30. Leg Lesser Yang Gall Bladder Channel

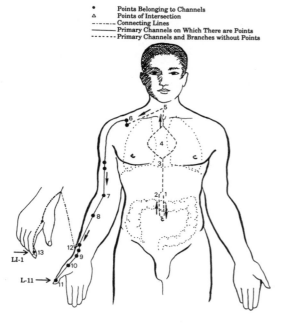

- • Points Belonging to Channels
- △ Points of Intersection
- —·—·— Connecting Lines
- ———— Primary Channels on Which There are Points
- ------- Primary Channels and Branches without Points

Figure 2-31. Arm Greater Yin Lung Channel

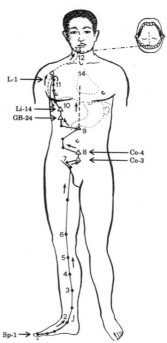

Figure 2-32. Leg Greater Yin Spleen Channel

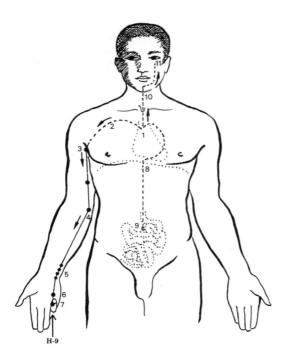

**Figure 2-33. Arm Lesser Yin
Heart Channel**

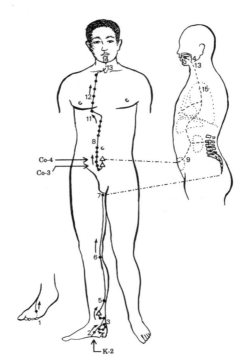

**Figure 2-34. Leg Lesser Yin
Kidney Channel**

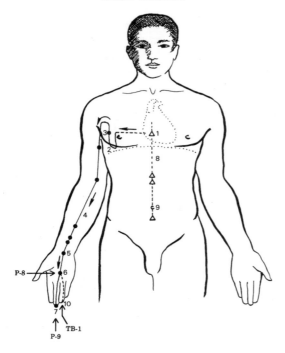

**Figure 2-35. Arm Absolute Yin
Pericardium Channel**

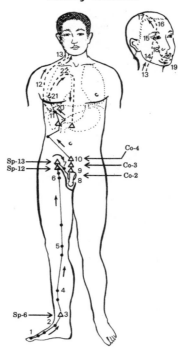

**Figure 2-36. Leg Absolute Yin
Liver Channel**

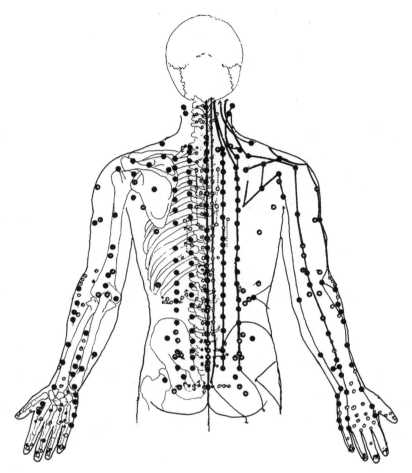

Figure 2-37. Primary Qi Channels and Acupuncture Cavities on the Back of the Body

Leg Greater Yin Spleen Channel (Zu Tai Yin Pi Jing, 足太陰脾經)(Figure 2-32)

Arm Lesser Yin Heart Channel (Shou Shao Yin Xin Jing, 手少陰心經) (Figure 2-33)

Leg Lesser Yin Kidney Channel (Zu Shao Yin Shen Jing, 足少陰腎經) (Figure 2-34)

Arm Absolute Yin Pericardium Channel (Shou Jue Yin Xin Bao Luo Jing, 手厥陰心包絡經)(Figure 2-35)

Leg Absolute Yin Liver Channel (Zu Jue Yin Gan Jing, 足厥陰肝經) (Figure 2-36)

3. From the above, you can see that one end of each channel connects to an extremity, and the other end connects with a different internal organ. In each channel, there are many acupuncture cavities through which the Qi condition

in each channel can be regulated. This is the basic theory of acupuncture.

4. There are thousands of secondary channels branching out from each primary; these lead the Qi to the surface of the skin and to the bone marrow. It is very similar to the artery and capillary system. Instead of blood, Qi is being distributed.

5. There are thirty-eight miscellaneous cavities (M-BW-1 to M-BW-38) on the sides of the vertebrae where the nerves branch out from the spinal cord (Figure 2-37). Stimulating these cavities properly can relax all the nerve junctions and also affect the Qi circulation in the Governing Vessel.

6. On each side of these cavities are two branches to the Yang Urinary Bladder channel. This channel runs straight down from the top of the head to the bottom of the feet, splitting into two parallel branches on the back (Figure 2-37). On the inner branch are cavities which are closely related to the health of the internal organs.

You do not have to remember all of these cavities and where they are located. We will list the cavities which are related to massage healing for back pain later, in chapter 6. This introduction is only to present the concepts. If you are interested in knowing more about these systems, please refer to an acupuncture book.[4]

Understanding the Central Energy System

1. The spine is the center of our Qi distribution system. From the spinal cord, through the nervous system that branches out to the entire body, we can feel and sense our body and its surroundings. Moreover, through this system, our mind is able to govern and control our body for any activity.

2. The spinal cord is part of the Thrusting Vessel in Chinese medicine, and connects the brain to the perineum. The Qi in this vessel is most activated in the midnight hours, while we are sleeping. This vessel is connected directly to the Qi residence or bioelectric battery, the Real Lower Dan Tian, located at the physical body's center of gravity.

3. As mentioned earlier, we have two brains, one is in our head and the other is in the gut. These two brains are connected with the spinal cord, and communicate with each other. The spinal cord is a highly electric conductive tissue (i.e., very low electric resistance). Therefore, even though physically there are two brains, in function they act as one single unit. **The upper brain generates an idea (i.e., EMF) and immediately the bioelectricity is supplied from the Real Lower Dan Tian, through the nervous system to the part of the body for action.**

4. Whenever there is a tightness or strain in the spine, the Qi distribution will be affected and could stagnate. Consequently, the nervous system will not function smoothly and efficiently. This means that communication between our brains and body will be slow or incomplete.

5. In order to have a smooth Qi supply to the nervous system, the spine must maintain its comfortable and healthy state. All of this depends on the health and strength of your torso muscles, which support the spine. When these muscles are weak or injured, the pressure on the joints of the spine will be increased, resulting in back pain.

6. Due to the abundant Qi supply circulating in the Thrusting and Governing Vessels, most of our blood cells are produced in the bone marrow of our spine and pelvic bones. White blood cells are the soldiers of our immune system. When there are plenty of healthy white blood cells, our immune system is strong and defensive capability is high. Moreover, when the Qi is abundant, each white blood cell will have the strength and power to destroy germs, bacteria and other unwelcome material intruding into our body. Qi is just like the food for the soldiers. If soldiers do not have plenty of food, their fighting capability will be low. Therefore, the most important key to strengthening our immune system is to keep this central energy system healthy, both physically and energetically.

7. In the entire torso, the muscles' condition in the lower back area is the most important. This is the only area where there is no strong support from the skeleton. The only skeletal support in this area is the lumbar vertebrae; this allows us to bow forward and bend sideways and backward slightly. Also because of this, the muscles in the lower back play an important role in supporting this area. When the muscles here are injured or weak due to degeneration, the pressure on the lumbar vertebrae will be increased, and pain will be generated. Therefore, in order to prevent lower back pain, the muscles in the waist area must be in good condition.

8. According to Chinese medicine, the kidney Qi channel runs from the kidneys through the lower back to the bottom of the foot. Whenever there is a tightness or pain in the lower back, the Qi status in the kidneys will be irregular, i.e., either too Yin or too Yang. When this happens, the function of the kidneys will be abnormal. A common problem as a person ages is lower back pain, often followed by kidney problems.

9. From the perspective of both Western and Eastern medicine, we know that whenever we eat, after the blood absorbs nutrients in the large and small intestines, the blood then passes through the liver. The liver, like a checking station, will filter the blood before the nutrients are distributed to the entire body through the blood circulatory system. During this process, acid is produced in the liver. This acid is then generally processed through the kidneys to the urinary system. That is why, when you get a physical check up, the doctor checks the pH value in your urine, to see if the acid is being taken away from your body normally. If the kidneys fail or are functioning under some sort of stress, the acid level in the body will rise. This acid will normally accumulate in the joints and become the well known form of arthritis called

gout. Naturally, the Qi level in the liver will also become abnormal, causing increased susceptibility to sickness.

10. According to Chinese medicine, the liver's condition is closely related to the heart. Whenever the Qi is too Yang in the liver, the heart will also become more Yang. Too much Yang in the heart can trigger a heart attack.

From the above discussion, you may already begin to see that the first and most essential key to maintaining health is to keep the torso strong, especially in the waist area. Next, you must know how to exercise the ligaments which connect the vertebrae joints. When these ligaments are strong and healthy, the spine is healthy. Spinal Qigong exercise is one of the martial Qigong practices which can lead you to this goal. In chapter 6, we will introduce these exercises.

References

1. "Anatomy of a Backache," *FDA Consumer,* April 1989.

2. "A Look at Disks," *The Baltimore Sun,* May 19, 1992.

3. "Outpatient Management of Low Back Pain," Judith A. Chase, *Orthopedic Nursing,* January/February 1992, Vol. 11/No. 1.

4. *Acupuncture—A Comprehensive Text*, Shanghai College of Traditional Medicine, Eastland Press, Chicago, 1981.

CHAPTER 3

What are the Possible Causes of Back Pain?

背疼的原因

3-1. Introduction

Back pain can be caused by overstretching or other trauma to the back muscles and/or tendons. It can also be caused by a tearing or inflammation of the ligaments in the spine. However, the most common and serious cause of back pain is spasm of the muscles in the lower back area brought on by spinal disease, injury or degeneration. Naturally, all of these problems can arise from many different circumstances. In this chapter, we will summarize the possible causes in Western terminology. Because lower back pain is the most common type of back pain, most of the research materials I have collected focus on this area.

3-2. The Different Possible Causes of Lower Back Pain

In order to have a clear understanding about lower back pain, we can envision that the spinal elements are structured as a "three-joint complex," with **a disc** and **two facet joints** at each level. If there is any change in one element, the other two will also be affected. When a person assumes a normal relaxed, standing position, the vertebral bodies will be loosely piled on top of each other. Whenever there is a disease which affects any one of the three elements, the intrinsic muscles will contract and develop protective splinting to prevent any microinstability that may occur, which can then result in ischemia (localized tissue anemia due to obstruction of the inflow of arterial blood) from prolonged contraction and begin to ache, lose tone, and eventually atrophy.[1]

Types of Pain

The prime symptom of spine problems is pain. Pain is the most common signal that the body uses to notify your brain about the problem of Qi imbalance or possible physical damage/injury to your body. Pain generated from structures other than the spinal cord or nerve roots can be classified as either local, referred, and muscular. If you are able to identify the type of pain you have, you may be able to better pinpoint the problem.

Local Pain[2]

Local pain usually results from the irritation of nerve endings at the site of the pathologic process. Local pain is usually steady and aching; it may occur off and on, particularly when the involved structure is moved. Local pain is commonly associated with tenderness to palpation or percussion. The site of local pain can be diagnosed relatively easier than other causes of back pain.

For example, metastatic tumors and osteoporotic collapse of a vertebral body can cause pain at the site of the lesion by irritating the nerve endings in the periosteum surrounding the vertebrae body. However, those metastatic tumors involving the vertebral body that do not upset the periosteum are usually painless. Other than the neck and lower back, tumors also often strike the thoracic area, and osteoporotic vertebral collapse also tends to affect the structurally weak thoracic vertebral bodies.

Intervertebral discs may also cause local pain when they compress nerve endings in the anulus fibrosus or posterior longitudinal ligament. Most spine pain from mechanical causes, such as a herniated disc, occur either in the neck or lower back because these structures are more mobile and more subject to injury.

The character of local pain is frequently helpful in diagnosis. Pain caused by lumbar muscle, ligamentous strain or herniated discs usually disappears when the patient lies down and the torso is relaxed. Herniated lumbar disc pain is often made worse by sitting and is relieved when standing or walking. However, on the contrary, the pain of spinal stenosis is often absent when lying or sitting, and occurs only when the patient walks. Vertebral metastases with or without epidural spinal cord compression cause pain. The pain is often more serious when lying and sometimes is relieved by sitting up. To ease the pain, many patients with spinal cord compression elect to sleep in a sitting position. Often, even if pain is absent when lying down, any movement such as turning over or getting up,may be particularly painful.

Referred Pain, Radicular Pain, and Funicular Pain[2]

Referred Pain. Referred pain is felt at a distance from the site of the local lesion, but not in the dermatomal distribution of a nerve root (radicular pain). Referred pain, like local pain, has a deep aching quality and is often associated with tender-

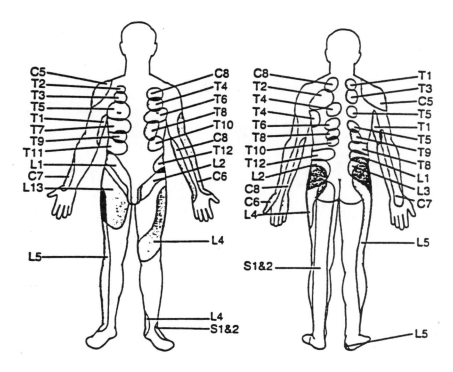

Figure 3-1. Sclerotomal Distribution of Pain

ness of subcutaneous tissues and muscles at the site of referral. Treating maneuvers that affect local pain usually have the same effect on referred pain. Referred pain produces a sclerotomal distribution of pain (Figure 3-1)[1]. Pain referred from pathologic abnormalities of the cervical spine often is either just medial to the scapula or over the lateral aspect of the arm. Pain referred from the lower back is usually appreciated in the buttocks and posterior thighs, although rarely below the knees. Pain from the upper lumbar spine is also often referred to the flank, groin, and anterior thigh. Pain also can be referred to the spine from lesions of thoracic or abdominal viscera, a prominent example being back pain from pancreatic carcinoma. Referred back pain from a visceral source is usually not worsened by positional changes, as is mechanical lower back pain.

Radicular Pain.[1 & 2] Injured spinal roots or an injured spinal cord can also produce, respectively, radicular or funicular pain. Radicular pain is the prime symptom of nerve root compression. Nerve roots are not usually pain-sensitive. However, chronic compression can lead to edema, and perhaps inflammation and demyelination. In this case, the root will become sensitive to stretching or compression. When compressed, the pain may be experienced only in the cutaneous distribution (dermatome) of the involved root or may be felt locally and deep in muscles that it supplies. Root pain is usually least severe in proper positions, in which the root compression is minimized. Naturally, the pain will become serious in positions that

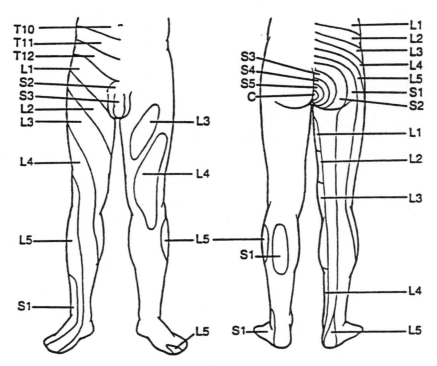

Figure 3-2. Radicular or Dermatomal Distribution of Pain

cause the root to be compressed or stretched. Root pain is usually worsened by increased intraspinal pressure due to coughing, sneezing, and straining.

Although similar, the pain distribution of radicular pain is not identical to referred pain (Figure 3-2)[1]. A common misconception is that referred pain radiates only as far down as the knee, and radicular pain radiates only below the knee. In fact, the only distinguishing feature between the two types of pain is in their quality. Referred pain is an aching or sore type of pain, while radicular pain is a sharp, lancinating, or burning type of pain.

Although the exact mechanism of nerve root compromise is not known, there are four known possible causes of radicular pain:

1. Direct mechanical compression of the nerve (neuritis).

2. Compression of the vasa nervorum, which produces a local anemia caused by mechanical obstruction of the blood supply (ischemia).

3. Venous obstruction.

4. Chemical irritation of the dural sleeve (i.e., the dura mater that covers the spinal cord), which causes inflammation (duritis). Dura mater is a tough, fibrous, whitish membrane (the outermost of the three membranes) that covers the brain and spinal cord.

Funicular Pain.[2] Funicular pain is caused by compression of the long tracts of the spinal cord. Normally, funicular pain is less sharp than radicular pain and is often described as a cold, unpleasant sensation in the extremity. Its distribution is more diffuse than that of radicular pain but like root pain is usually worsened by movements that stretch the cord (e.g., neck flexion or straight leg raising) or that increase intraspinal pressure.

Muscle Pain.[2] Muscle pain occurs when paravertebral muscle spasm occurs due to an injury to or structural abnormality of the spine. Sustained contraction of paravertebral muscles causes chronic aching pain which is usually felt lateral to the midline of the neck or back. Palpation of painful muscles is a common diagnosis method to reveal evidence of spasm and tenderness. Often when areas of extreme sensitivity (trigger points) are palpated, the pain may be felt not only locally in the muscle but also may be referred to distant structures. These trigger points are considered as the causes underlying many myofascial pain syndromes of the neck and back without structural abnormalities of the spine.

Risk Factors[3]

In the same environment, some people get sick more easily than others because their immune system is not as strong. Similarly, many people have a greater chance of developing back pain than others. The reasons for this are the "roots" of this type of pain. If you do not study these reasons, but simply try to track down the causes of the symptoms, then even if you find relief, it is very likely that the problem will recur. Therefore, the best way of solving back pain problems and preventing them from occurring again is to find these roots. Next, we will examine the possible roots, or risk factors, which may cause back pain problems.

Physical Degeneration[3]

We cannot stop our physical degeneration, but we can slow down this degenerating process by providing proper care to our body. According to Chinese Qigong, to slow down our aging process, we must maintain the strength our physical body (Yang) and also learn how to increase the storage of inner energy in our Qi body (Yin). Normally, the health of our physical body can be achieved through physical exercises (physical Qigong), and the storage of our Qi in the Lower Dan Tian (human bioelectric battery) can be obtained from correct breathing and meditation. When these Yin and Yang sides of our body are cultivated, then health and longevity can be expected.

When we age, the first things that degenerate in our body are the muscles and tendons. Muscles reach their peak capacity by age 20, then decline without proper exercise. When our muscles and tendons are degenerating and weakening, the body's motor capacity goes down. Consequently, the pressure between the joints of our body increases and the degeneration of the joints speeds up. This degeneration process is even greater in the spine, which supports our body's weight and activity.

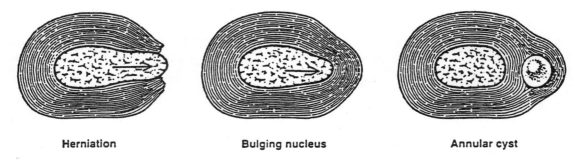

| Herniation | Bulging nucleus | Annular cyst |

Figure 3-3. The Nucleus Can Herniate or an Annular "Cyst" Can Bulge

The degeneration or deterioration of a part of the spine, especially the lower back, may result from a gradual wearing down of bone or soft connective tissue. It can also result from a reduction in the circulation of blood, which brings oxygen and other nutrients to the area. Degeneration is most likely to occur in the disc (cushion between the bones—vertebrae) or in the cartilage of the facet joints (joints between the vertebrae). In fact, both disc and joint disease are eventually present together.[1] **"Degenerative lumbar spondylosis"** refers to both. Therefore, degenerative disc disease can lead to degenerative joint disease and vice versa. When both the disc and the joint become involved, the pain is difficult to separate clinically.

Disc degeneration begins in the early 20s. Though discs in babies are about 90 percent water, by age 70 fluid loss reduces the water content to 70 percent, flattening the discs. Because discs constitute 25 percent of the spine's length, as the discs become flatter and less elastic, people lose height. In fact, most of us can expect to be about a half inch to two inches shorter in old age.

In addition, when discs deteriorate, they can crack and slip outward (**herniate**), tear, or flatten, causing excessive movement and irritation of the cartilage at the facet joints. The nucleus pulposus changes into fibrocartilage from the second decade on.[1] The loss of elasticity allows shearing forces to cross the disc unopposed. In addition, annular fibers can undergo localized myxomatous (degeneration caused by the presence of a benign tumor). This can lead to an osmotic gradient with the formation of a cyst within the annulus. This cyst can slowly enlarge and produce atraumatic disc bulging with consequent clinical signs and symptoms (Figure 3-3).

One or more discs might actually flatten, causing collapse of the vertebral column. When discs are flattened, they lose their ability to act as shock absorbers, putting greater stress on supporting ligaments, causing back pain. Pain can also result from the narrowing of the spinal canal (**stenosis**), which results in increased pressure on the nerves that branch out from the spinal cord.

In addition, as we age, various degrees of wear and tear on the spine may cause inflammation. This is commonly referred to as **degenerative arthritis** or **spondylitis**. If the degeneration is mild, no symptoms may appear. However, arthritis can destroy cartilage in the spine and cause bone overgrowth (spurs)(Figure 3-4).

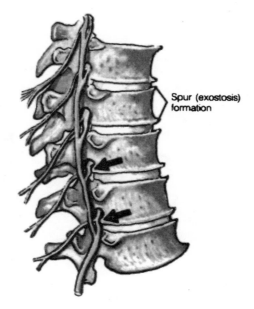

Spur (exostosis)
formation

Arrows indicate bone spurs
impinging on spinal nerves

Figure 3-4. Spinal Nerve Irritation Due to Exostosis (Bony Overgrowth)
(© Anatomical Chart Co., Skokie, IL.)

Another degenerative disease frequently affecting the back and causing back pain is **osteoporosis** (Figure 3-5). Osteoporosis is a condition in which bones become porous and susceptible to crushing or fracture. Though both men and women lose bone density after age 35, the disease appears most often in women past menopause.

Spinal joints are also affected by various forms of arthritis. One type that most of us will experience if we live long enough is degenerative joint disease, or **osteoarthritis**. The cartilage that cushions joints gradually breaks down, resulting in back pain and stiffness, especially in the morning. Osteoarthritis may appear as early as the 20s and 30s, though without symptoms, and nearly everybody has it by age 70.

In many cases of arthritis, pain that begins in the morning upon arising from sleep improves throughout the day with activity. Because the nerves that branch out from the spinal cord conduct impulses to all parts of the body, pressure on one or more nerves may cause pain that radiates into the hip and down the leg (**sciatica**) or tingling or numbness of an arm or leg. In more serious cases, there may be interference with bowel and bladder function, or, if nerves in the neck are compressed, difficulty speaking or respiratory problems.

Spinal osteophytosis, a normal function of aging, is produced by traction of the spinal ligaments on the periosteum of the vertebral bodies. It is not related to degenerative lumbar spondylosis.[1]

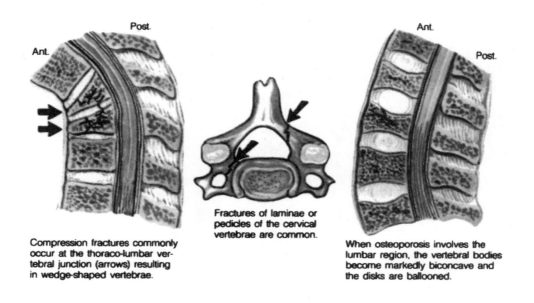

Compression fractures commonly occur at the thoraco-lumbar vertebral junction (arrows) resulting in wedge-shaped vertebrae.

Fractures of laminae or pedicles of the cervical vertebrae are common.

When osteoporosis involves the lumbar region, the vertebral bodies become markedly biconcave and the disks are ballooned.

Figure 3-5. Osteoporosis
(© Anatomical Chart Co., Skokie, IL.)

In spinal osteophytosis, the disc spaces are well preserved. The condition appears to be worse on the right side, probably due to inhibition of spur formation by the pulsating aorta along the left side. Some 90 percent of men older than 50 have some of these traction osteophytes in the lumbar area.

When spinal osteophytosis is excessive, it may represent a *forme fruste* of **diffuse idiopathic skeletal hyperostosis** (DISH), an ossifying diathesis of ligaments and tendons throughout the patient's body. DISH begins with ossification of the anterior longitudinal ligament of the dorsal spine, and then spreads to the cervical and lumbar spine. It is associated with widespread osteoarthritis as well as spurs where the ligaments and tendons attach to bone (**enthesopathy**). DISH is typically found in middle-aged men, 80 percent of whom appear to have adult-onset diabetes. It is also seen as a side effect of isotretinoin (Accutane) and excessive fluorine intake.

Degenerative spondylolisthesis is a condition where there is a forward slippage of one vertebra over another, usually of a lumbar vertebra on the vertebra below it, or upon the sacrum. Also called spondyloptosis. It is caused by subluxation of degenerated joints. Spondylolisthesis almost always occurs at L4-5 (Figure 3-6).

From the above summary, we can see that the most common symptom of physical degeneration of the spine is an aching back. It is believed that failure to develop adequate bone mass during youth, lack of exercise, and a diet low in calcium and other nutrients (i.e., poor physical fitness) may be contributing factors.

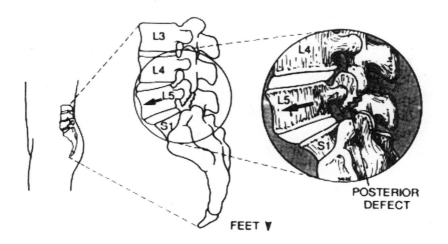

FEET ▼

POSTERIOR
DEFECT

Figure 3-6. Spondyloisthesis

Poor Life Styles

One of the most common and important root sources of sickness is the life style we live. Unfortunately, this factor is greatly ignored by the general public until the start of a problem. If we look at Eastern and Western concepts of health, we can clearly see that one of their main differences is that Chinese medicine gives serious attention to the prevention of sickness, while Western medicine emphasizes healing after the symptoms of sickness appear physically. Qigong developed from the motivation to maintain health and longevity. It is also because of this that the Chinese have paid more attention to observing the relationship between natural Qi and human Qi. From this awareness, many Qigong practices were initiated and blended into daily life. Since then, the ways of healthy living have been passed down from generation to generation for more than four thousand years.

If we calm down our mind, we can see a great difference between today's life styles and those of people living a century ago. Because of the fast development of science in this century, and despite the great benefits such development has brought us, our life style has significantly changed and become less dependent on natural cycles, thus removing us from the natural Dao, or "way of life," to which our evolution has suited us. It is because of this new life style, and the extremely short time in which we have had to adapt to it, that our body can have difficulties adapting to our environment. Therefore, many health problems can occur. The following are a few examples of such difficulties:

1. In the last fifty years, we have discovered a rapid increase in the number of cases of cancer. For example, it is estimated that 10 percent of women today may experience the pain of breast cancer. If we analyze the reason, we may conclude that this may be a result of the heavy energetic and material pollution we have created in the last few decades. However, if we calm down and

ponder more deeply, we can see that we have ignored another important factor of this for this occurrence—our life styles have changed.

Traditionally, even just forty years ago, most women got married when they were young (often in their late teens). Due to lack of knowledge and poor reproductive medicine, on average women were pregnant at a younger age and more often than they are today. Before this century, a woman would carry an average of ten babies in her lifetime.

Next, from a Chinese Qigong and medical standpoint, we must understand that men are generally more muscular, bigger in size, and physically more powerful than women. There are only two places where a woman is normally larger than a man physically—the hips and breasts. The reason for this is that women have evolved bigger muscles in the hip area to support the baby's extra weight, and the bone structure of the pelvis is specialized for passing a child through the birth canal. Moreover, the breast area is more developed than in men because this place produces milk for the baby. In order to produce enough milk to nourish the baby, the Qi in the breast area is normally highly abundant. From the baby's sucking of milk, the baby absorbs both nutrients and Qi from the mother. Therefore, between mother and baby, there is a spiritual communication and Qi balance during this feeding process.

However, since now we can control reproduction, most women today will carry no more than two or three babies. Moreover, because of the convenience of bottle feeding, the spiritual communication and Qi exchange process is missing. Therefore, there is a great quantity of under-utilized Qi stored in women's breasts today. If a woman does not practice Qigong arm exercises correctly and lead the excess Qi away from the breast area, the imbalance of Qi in the breast may result in the physical deformity that is breast cancer. From a Qigong point of view, this problem can become more significant, since today's women do not exercise their arms as much as they used to. The arm exercises are the crucial keys of leading the accumulated Qi away from the breast area. Furthermore, breast feeding is able to trigger increased hormone production and reduce the risk of breast cancer.

2. It was reported in May, 1996 that sperm counts in human males have been dropping significantly and steadily in the last two decades.[5] This implies that the human race could be facing a disastrous reproductive crisis in the not so far off future. The data has been linked to a buildup in the environment of commonly used chemicals that some scientists believe disrupt the hormone systems controlling reproduction and development in humans.

However, again we have ignored the most important consideration; the change in our life style. All human life styles in the past developed under the influence of nature. For example, since electricity was not yet discovered, our sleeping habits were influenced by the sun's rising and setting. Normally, a person in ancient times would go to bed just a couple of hours after sunset, and would wake up not long after sunrise. Therefore, the Qi circulation in our body has been significantly influenced by this natural cycle. During the day time, most of the Qi was led by the mind to the muscles for daily physical activity (Yang activity), while in the night, the physical body rested during sleep, and the Qi circulated inward to nourish the bone marrow, the brain, and the sexual organs through the spinal cord (i.e., Thrusting Vessel)(Yin activity).[6] Normally, this process and change from Yang to Yin takes about three hours, assuming deep physical rest and sleep. Therefore, according to the understanding of Chinese Qigong, the Qi heavily and actively circulates in the central energy conduit (i.e., the spinal cord or Thrusting Vessel) at around midnight.

Now, let us take a look of today's life style. Ordinarily, people do not go to bed until after midnight. That means that, when we go to bed, we have already missed the natural timing of the brain's nourishment, as well as sperm production. This natural timing of the sperm production has developed after millions of years of evolution. Naturally, it is not going to be easy to adjust to our new life style in just a few short decades.

3. Today, we commonly experience more knee problems than we did forty years ago. What is surprising is that this has happened to both the young and the old. Human legs are much bigger and more powerful than arms, simply because we have walked for a million years by using our legs. After our body developed to this stage through walking, suddenly in the last forty years, automobiles have become popular. We now travel almost everywhere by car, short trips as well as long. Walking from one place to another has become a painful process. Because of this, our knees have degenerated rapidly in the last forty years. A child spends many hours per week watching television or playing video games, then grows up to travel almost everywhere by car. Is it any wonder that our knees are not what they used to be?

4. Similarly, because of the absence of physical activity or exercise of our torso, our spine has rapidly undergone a general deterioration in the last few generations. This has resulted in many spine problems. Machines have replaced human labor to the benefit of many, but have also destroyed natural body structures which evolved over millions of years.

In addition to the above four examples, there are many other problems caused by today's new life style. Of course, in many ways I believe that we should continue to develop science, technology and medicine because of the wonderful benefits it brings to the world. However, the consequences of such developments are not without the potential for harm. We must pay more attention to these consequences as we consider what path our scientific development should take. For example, many kinds of electro-magnetic radiation (radio waves, microwaves, etc.) pass through our body today at various levels of intensity. These human-made electromagnetic waves were non-existent as recently as the beginning of this century. How do these waves affect our body? We have already discussed how our body, as a bioelectric organism has an electromagnetic field that can be influenced by the surrounding electromagnetic field of the planet. How much will the energy circulating in our body be influenced because of the electric light-created night shift, or even the time dilating effects of jet lag. Therefore, we can see that it is our responsibility to urge our governments to give this area of study its proper attention. Only then will humanity really obtain the full benefits of scientific development.

Now, let us analyze and summarize the possible factors resulting from our current life style which may be the causes of back pain:

1. **Imbalance of Torso.** Since the spine is a masterfully balanced piece of architecture, if there is an influence which is able to constantly disrupt the balance of our torso, the strain on one side of the torso can be worse than on the other side. Back pain can be a consequence of this imbalance.

   For example, shoes with high heels can make you constantly adjust your torso from leaning forward. This can generate imbalance-induced stress in the spine.

2. **Long Periods of Sitting or Standing.** It is believed that many cases of lower back pain are caused by stress in the muscles and ligaments that support the spine. Long periods of sitting and standing can make the torso muscles fatigue and lose the strength to support the body's balance or upright posture. If a weak muscle is overburdened it can go into spasm (sudden, involuntary contractions that can be excruciatingly painful), affecting the whole network of back muscles. When this happens, back pain can result. This possibility is more significant for people whose physical fitness is poor. Often, even after the muscle spasm subsides, the muscle remains tighter than it was before the injury. This will limit movement in related joints and make new injury more likely.

3. **Poor Postures or Improper Body Movements.** Poor postures in sitting or standing can generate an imbalance in the torso. This will affect the structure of the spine. Normally, this problem can result from poor posture activities like watching too much television, working for too long on a computer, or poor sleeping habits (i.e., on stomach, soft mattress).

   Common spine problems resulting from poor postures are scoliosis (Figure 3-7) or lordosis (Figure 3-8), which are caused by the uneven narrowing of one area of the discs.

   Sometimes, improper body movements can cause damage to the spine. For example, a sudden twist or fall can bring on muscle spasm. A spasm immobilizes the muscles over the injured area, possibly acting as a kind of splint to protect muscles or joints from further damage. Improper body movements usually occur while you are engaged in physical labor or sports.

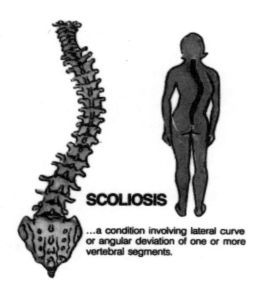

SCOLIOSIS

...a condition involving lateral curve or angular deviation of one or more vertebral segments.

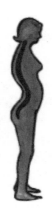

LORDOSIS

...an exaggeration of the posterior concavity of the spine characteristic of the lumbar region. It is also called "swayback" indicating extreme anterior curvature of the lumbar spine.

Figure 3-7. Scoliosis
(© Anatomical Chart Co., Skokie, IL.)

Figure 3-8. Lordosis
(© Anatomical Chart Co., Skokie, IL.)

4. **Poor Physical Fitness.** If you are in poor physical condition, especially in the abdominal muscles, you cannot support the spine properly, and strains or sprains can be recurrent. The fact is that it doesn't take much to overstretch (strain) a muscle or put a small tear (sprain) in a ligament. The medical word for backaches arising from either of these conditions is **lumbosacral strain** (or **sprain**).

   The main cause of poor physical conditioning is lack of exercise, or improper exercise. Too little exercise is not effective in building up the strength of the torso. Too much exercise can also be harmful, especially when the muscles are in a fatigued condition and can be easily injured. Good exercise for healthy physical fitness is exercise that is able to build up both the strength and endurance of the muscles, tendons and ligaments.

5. **Obesity.** Bad eating habits or poor food choices can cause weight problems. This can worsen if the person also fails to exercise. Obesity increases both the weight supported by the spine and the pressure on the discs within the spine, therefore generating spine problem more easily than in other people.

6. **Types of Jobs.** Jobs that involve bending and twisting, or the lifting of heavy objects repeatedly, especially when the loads are beyond a worker's strength, are no better for the back than are sedentary jobs. Certain occupations, such as truck driving or nursing, are particularly hard on the back. The truck driver must contend with sitting for long periods (actually worse for the back than standing), the vibration of the vehicle, and lifting and straining at the

end of the day when muscles are fatigued and more susceptible to damage. It has been shown that the dorsal muscles become easily fatigued when subjected to seated vibration.[7] In fact, truck driving ranks first in workmen's compensation cases for lower back pain.

7. **Sports or Gymnastics.** Football, gymnastics and other strenuous sports can also damage the lower back. In addition, degeneration may also occur in younger people, such as ballet dancers or athletes, where required movements repeatedly place extreme pressure on one or more parts of the spine. A curvature of the spine (**scoliosis**) may cause the vertebral joints to move in abnormal ways leading to more pronounced degeneration.

8. **Smoking.**[7] An 18 percent greater mean disc degeneration score in all levels of the lumbar spine has been reported in smokers as compared with nonsmokers. Over-consumption of alcohol may also be involved in disc degeneration.

Genetic Predisposition

A particularly distressing type of arthritis is **ankylosing spondylitis (Figure 3-9).** The lower back and sacroiliac joints become stiff and swollen. Muscles spasm and back pain may be so severe that bending over is the only way to find relief. If untreated, in some cases the inflamed spinal joints may fuse, preventing the individual from straightening up. The disease affects more men than women, usually starting between the ages of twenty and forty, though it can begin as early as age ten. The cause is unknown, but it is believed that some people may be **genetically susceptible** to this disorder. Posture-maintaining exercises, hot baths, painkillers and nonsteroidal anti-inflammatory drugs may help relieve symptoms.

In addition, those people whose height is above average can also experience back pain more frequently than those of average height. This is simply because it is harder for them to bend their upper body without putting more stress or strain on the lower back. The worst part of life for these very tall people is using mass transportation, utilities, clothes, machines, etc. which are designed for people of average height. The necessity of living their life in a world that is two feet too short can be depressing both mentally and physically.

It is also a fact that normally, our two legs are not the same length. If the difference is over a quarter inch, the imbalance to the torso can cause muscle spasms, especially if you have to walk for a long distance.

Mental (Spiritual) Excitement or Depression

Mental (spiritual) excitement or depression can occur if you are emotionally disturbed. For example, too much excitement or sadness can create strain in the torso, and therefore cause back pain. You should learn how to regulate your mind and maintain your emotions in a neutral and harmonious state.

Another common factor in depression is work dissatisfaction. According to reports, individuals who stated that they "hardly ever" enjoyed their job tasks were 2.5 times more likely to report back injury than were those who "almost always"

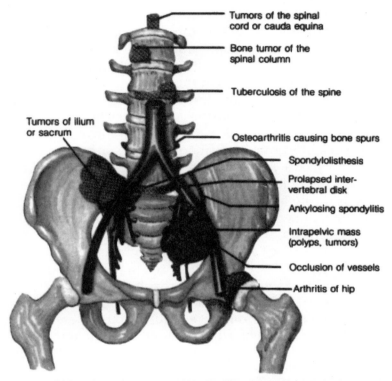

Tumors of the spinal cord or cauda equina

Bone tumor of the spinal column

Tuberculosis of the spine

Tumors of ilium or sacrum

Osteoarthritis causing bone spurs

Spondylolisthesis

Prolapsed inter-vertebral disk

Ankylosing spondylitis

Intrapelvic mass (polyps, tumors)

Occlusion of vessels

Arthritis of hip

Not all lower back pains are caused by protruding disks or extruded nucleus pulposus. Shown above (diagrammatically) are ten other causes that the examining physician must consider as possibilities in the diagnosis.

Figure 3-9. Ankylosing Spondylitis
(© Anatomical Chart Co., Skokie, IL.)

enjoyed their job task.[7] When this happens, emotional depression can be generated which could result in back pain.

Causes:

Mechanical Lower Back Pain. This means there is a biomechanical dysfunction. This is the number one cause of most complaints of lower back pain. Pain occurs when there is an alteration of one or more of the vertebrae and/or joints. This type usually creates pain with certain movements.

Muscular strains are commonly associated with back pain problems. This can also happen when back muscles are overloaded or fatigued. This may create a dull, aching pain that hurts in any position. Normally, it is not accompanied by leg pain and it generally heals in seven to ten days.

Ligamentous sprains can also occur when ligaments are overloaded. This condition generally takes two to four weeks to heal. Normally, there is no leg pain with this condition either.

Disc Problems. When a disc receives excessive or uneven pressure, pain can be generated. This condition will usually produce leg pain and sensations such as numbness, tingling and muscle weakness. Before reading this section further, it is advised that you first review the last chapter for a discussion of the structure and function of the discs. This will provide you with a better foundation for understanding the problems which can originate from in the discs.

Note that disc metabolism is very slow and anaerobic. It is the movement of the nucleus pulposus anteriorly during extension and posteriorly during flexion that allows for the flow of nutrients into the disc. If we do not move the spine or do not know how to move the vertebrae joint area smoothly and softly, the flow of the nutrients and fluid required for healthy discs will be deficient. Therefore, damage to the spine can easily be triggered. In fact, the Qigong exercises which will be introduced in this book mainly focus on such spine joint movements. This is a significant key to healing. Next, let us examine the general disc problems which have commonly been seen in medical spine treatments.

Disc Prolapse (Herniated Disc). Actually, the term "slipped disc" is inaccurate because the disc doesn't slip at all. A disc is anchored in place and does not, in fact, fall out of place. Because many people are familiar with the term "slipped" disc, this problem is mistakenly believed to be the chief cause of most lower back pain. But in fact, slipped discs are responsible for only five percent to ten percent of the cases. In some cases, the tough tissues (nucleus pulposus) that contain the disc are weakened or degenerated due to injuries or aging, allowing the soft gel-like center (annulus fibrosus) to protrude. Generally, physicians prefer the terms "herniated disc" or "prolapsed disc" to describe what happens when a disc bulges out or ruptures.[8]

As mentioned, before a prolapse of the nucleus pulposus can occur, the patient must have already experienced circumferential tears that weaken the annulus enough so that the next traumatic episode produces a radial tear (Figure 3-10). In most of these cases, this results in a bulging disc. The exception occurs when the radial tear extends through Sharpey's fibers. As a result, there is a herniation that can separate as a free fragment. In summary the nucleus can herniate or bulge, or an annular "cyst" can bulge (Figure 3-3).[1] If the protrusion presses on a nerve root, pinching it against the bone, the result is pain in the area of the body served by that nerve.[8 & 9]

Disc prolapse is less likely to occur during the day because the disc becomes more elastic as its water content decreases. In the work place, however, any benefit from the extra elasticity is canceled by the fatigue that progressively increases throughout the day.[1]

The protruded part of the disc does not slip back into place. Scar tissue forms around the protrusion and walls it in. If the outer tissues continue to be stressed, they will weaken further and, in time, the slightest activity—a sneeze or cough—may cause the disc to burst through its capsule, or rupture.[9]

As might be expected, pain from disc disease can rank pretty high on the pain index. To make matters worst, if a nerve root is irritated in any one place, it tends to become irritable along its whole length. A ruptured disc that presses on nerve roots

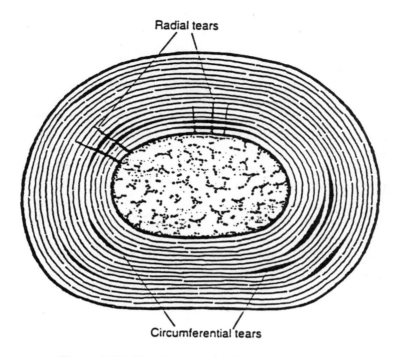

Radial tears

Circumferential tears

Figure 3-10. The Axial View of Annular Tears

in the lower back (lower lumbar or high sacral areas) causes **sciatica**, a condition in which sharp, shooting pains begin in the buttock and run down the back of the thigh and the inside of the leg to the foot. Tingling, numbness and weakness may follow. If the pressure on the nerve root is not relieved, the leg muscles will eventually waste away, or atrophy.[9]

When sciatica occurs, doctors can usually pinpoint the specific nerve root of roots that are compressed in most cases by carefully examining the strength of individual muscles and deep tendon reflexes, and by noting where there's loss of sensation. Conservative treatment such as strict bed rest, anti-inflammatory medication, and muscle relaxants often relieve the acute symptoms. In intractable cases, surgery may be necessary to relieve pressure on the nerve root.[9]

Fracture. Any bone fracture in the spine can cause a sharp pain. Whenever there is a fracture in the spine, the nerves in the surrounding area will be irritated and cause the muscles and tendons to spasm. Normally, this kind of back pain will last until the fracture of the bone is completely healed.

Lumbar Strain and Lumbar Spondylosis. Back pain can be caused due to lumbar strain. The patient can decrease the strain on the discs by tightening the abdominal muscles to transform the abdominal cavity into a semi-rigid cylinder. If degenerative disease causes intrinsic muscle atrophy, extension is achieved almost exclusively from the glutei. This puts more traction (i.e., pulling) on the greater trochanter (one of the two prominences on the upper part of the femur). As a result, there is a higher incidence of bursitis of the greater trochanter in degenerative lumbar spondylosis. Spondylosis is an abnormal immobility and fixation of a vertebral joint caused from narrowing of disc space and arthritis changes of facet joint (facet arthritis).[1]

Spinal Stenosis. Degenerative spinal stenosis occurs when facet osteophytes narrow the canal posteriorly and disc bulging narrows the canal anteriorly.

Spondylolisthesis and Spondylolysis. Spondylolisthesis is a case when there is a forward slippage of one vertebra over another, usually of a lumbar vertebra on the vertebra below it, or upon the sacrum. It is also called spondyloptosis (Figure 3-6).

Spondylolysis is when there is a breaking down or destruction of a vertebra.

Severe Scoliosis and Kyphosis. Scoliosis is a rotary lateral curvature of the spine (Figure 3-7). When the case becomes serious, back pain can be generated.

Kyphosis is similar but different. Kyphosis is when there is an abnormal, rearward increase in the curvature of the thoracic spine (Figure 3-11). It is also called hunchback or humpback.

Lumbar Hyperlordosis. Hyperlordosis (sway-back) is a well-recognized cause of lower back pain. This pain occurs when the anterior longitudinal ligament and facet joints are stretched. Hyperlordosis often develops during pregnancy because of poor abdominal tone. It is aggravated by wearing high-heeled shoes and standing for prolonged periods.

Normally, flexion of the lumbar spine proceeds from L1 sequentially to S1, with each functional unit flexing 8 to 10 degrees, totaling 45 degrees of lumbar flexion. Simultaneous pelvic rotation via hip flexion increases the flexion to 135 degree. When straightening, one derotates the pelvis first.

Rotation of the lumbar spine occurs only from T12-L1 and L4-5. In addition, L4-5 is not protected by the pelvis or the pelvic ligaments, as is L5-S1. Therefore, it is subjected to the greatest load-bearing stress and is most often the first disc involved in acute disc herniation.[1]

Bacterial Endocarditis. Endocarditis is an inflammation of the endocardium. Endocardium is the thin, endothelial (i.e., thin layer of flat cells that lines serous cavities, lymph vessels, and blood vessels), serous membrane that lines the interior of the heart.

Bacterial Endocarditis is an endocarditis due to bacteria or other microorganisms, causing deformity of the valve leaflets; it may be acute, usually caused by pyogenic organisms such as staphylococci or subacute (chronic), usually due to *Streptococcus viridans* or *Streptococcus faecalis*. These bacteria usually attack the intestines.

Osteomyelitis. Osteomyelitis is a type of bone infection that affects the metaphyseal regions of the long bones. In the United States, 50 percent of the cases are caused by *Staphyloccus aureus*. Salmonella infections are commonly found in individuals with sickle cell disease. Spinal lesions are commonly caused by tuberculosis or gram-negative organisms. These are organisms that cannot be detected using standard dying techniques.

Osteoporosis. As mentioned earlier, osteoporosis is a degenerative disease frequently affecting the back and causing back pain. Osteoporosis is a disease of the

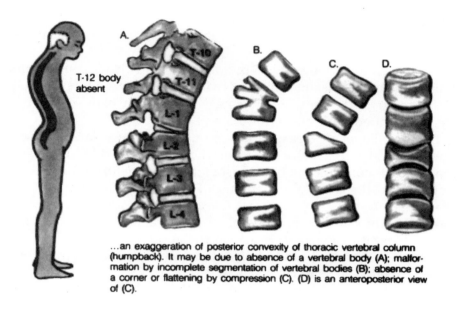

...an exaggeration of posterior convexity of thoracic vertebral column (humpback). It may be due to absence of a vertebral body (A); malformation by incomplete segmentation of vertebral bodies (B); absence of a corner or flattening by compression (C). (D) is an anteroposterior view of (C).

Figure 3-11. Kyphosis
(© Anatomical Chart Co., Skokie, IL.)

bones due to deficiency of bone matrix, occurring most frequently in post-menopausal women.

Paraspinous Abscess. A localized collection of pus in the spine, formed by tissue disintegration and surrounding by an inflamed area.

Ankylosing Spondylitis. An abnormally immobilized joint caused by inflammation of one or more vertebrae (Figure 3-9).

Inflammatory Bowel Disease. Some arthritis associated with inflammatory bowel disease can cause back pain.

Reiter's Syndrome (RS). Reiter's Syndrome is a symptom complex consisting of urethritis, conjunctivitis, arthritis, and mucocutaneous lesions. Recurrences or chronicity occur in more than one-half of the patients. Its etiology remains unknown.

Psoriatic Arthritis. Arthritis which is associated with psoriasis. Psoriasis is a chronic skin disease characterized by reddish patches covered with silvery scales, occurring most often on the knees, elbows, scalp, and trunk.

Exostosis. Exostosis is the case where there is a bone growth on the surface of a bone. This can occur if there is an arthritis-destroying cartilage in the spine causing bone overgrowth (Figure 3-4)(**spurs**). When this happens, the spinal nerve can be impinged or irritated which causes pain.

Lymphoma. Any of a group of malignant diseases originating in the lymphoreticular system, usually in the lymph nodes.

Multiple Myeloma. Disease characterized by the appearance of scattered malignant tumors in various bones of the body; it is generally associated with the production of abnormal globulins and the presence of Bence Jones protein in the urine.

Multiple myeloma occurs mostly in persons in the sixth to eighth decade of life and affects males more often than females. Also called myelomatosis; plasma cell myeloma.

Metastatic Carcinoma. Metastatic carcinoma is a malignant cellular tumor which is derived from epithelial tissue and tends to invade surrounding tissues and/or spread to other parts of the body by metastasis, eventually causing death.

Primary Bone Tumors. Primary tumors on bones.

Paget's Disease. Paget's Disease is a bone disease of unknown cause which is characterized by localized areas of bone destruction followed by replacement with overdeveloped, light, soft, porous bone associated with deformities, such as thickening of portions of the skull and bending of weight-bearing bones. Also called osteitis deformans.

Abdominal Aortic Aneurysm. Abdominal aortic aneurysm is a circumscribed sac-like bulging generating an aortic vessel at the abdominal area.

Gastrointestinal Disease. A kind of disease which is related to the stomach and intestines. Also called gastroenteric diseases.

Prostatitis. Inflammation of the prostate and the bladder.

Endometriosis. An abnormal condition in which the uterine mucous membrane invades other tissues in the pelvic cavity; the uterus and ovaries are the most common sites; other areas include the intestines, umbilicus, bladder and ureters.

Chronic Pelvic Inflammatory Disease (PID). An inflammation in the pelvic cavity, especially of the female genital organs.

Pyelonephritis. Inflammation of the kidneys, especially the renal pelvis. Also called pyelitis.

Psychogenic Pain Syndrome. A set of signs and symptoms in pain generated from the mind that appear with reasonable consistency.

Cauda Equina Syndrome. Cauda Equina is a large protrusion which may press on the nerves that branch off the end of the spinal cord, causing back pain, loss of sensation in the buttocks, thighs or genital organs, and bowel and bladder disturbances. When this, or any other symptoms of nerve root pressure occurs, help should be sought immediately.[1]

References

1. "Acute and Chronic Lower Back Pain: How to Pinpoint Its Cause and Make the Diagnosis," Burton Sack, *Modern Medicine,* Vol. 50, September 1992.

2. "Section Fifteen/Mechanical Lesions of the Spine and Related Structures," Jerome B. Posner, M.D., Excerpted from *Cecil Textbook of Medicine, Vol. 2,* 1988.

3. "Outpatient Management of Lower Back Pain," Judith A. Chase, *Orthopaedic Nursing,* January/February 1992, Vol 11/No. 1.

4. *Degeneration Problems of the Back*, NIAMS, August, 1992.

5. "Sperm Count Drop: Is It Just Bad Data?" Richard Saltus, *Boston Globe,* May 20, 1996.

6. *Muscle/Tendon Changing and Marrow/Brain Washing Chi Kung*, Jwing-Ming Yang, YMAA, 1989.

7. "Perspective on Lower Back Pain," Ian K.Y. Tsang, MB, FRCP(C), *Current Science,* 1993.

8. "A Look at Discs," *The Baltimore Sun,* May 19, 1992.

9. *Back Talk: Advice for Suffering Spines*, Evelyn Zamula, FDA Consumer, April 1989.

CHAPTER 4

How Does Western Medicine Treat Back Pain?

背疼的原因

4-1. Introduction

Before the development of modern medicine, when a person suffered back pain, it was treated with rest, massage, heat, or gentle movements until the pain subsided. Later after modern medicine became popular in the second half of this century, pain killing drugs, ice to reduce inflammation, and rest were heavily utilized. However, during the last decade or so, as we have gained a better understanding of the anatomic structure of the spine and learned more about the possible causes of these problems, and as the price of clinical medical treatments has gone up, a new paradigm for treatment and experiments has emerged. Here are some of the facts that have been discovered by modern Western medicine according to recent reports.[1 & 2]

1. Back pain is one of the diseases which is most difficult for the physician to diagnose. It is often troublesome to treat, and always lasts longer than the patient and his care givers would like.

2. Most back pain is caused by muscles that go into spasm. The cause of the spasm of the muscles can be either non-related or closely related to spine problems.

3. The majority of back pain problems are self-correcting and resolved within a few weeks.

4. Lower back pain and disability does not progressively increase with age, nor does it correspond to the age-related changes of disc degeneration.

5. There is little difference in the effectiveness of any type of treatment for

lower back pain, and there is no scientific evidence that any one treatment is any better than others

6. Chronic lower back pain is a completely different syndrome than acute lower back pain and is treated differently.

7. According to a new study in *The New England Journal of Medicine*, two days of bed rest are enough for most acute backaches. More than two days' rest can further weaken muscles.[3]

8. The traditional explanation for chronic back pain, the "slipped disc," actually accounts for fewer than 5 percent of back injuries. In fact, with the increased use of CAT scans (please see next section for more information about CAT scans), doctors are now finding that many people, if not most, have disc abnormalities, which **don't** contribute directly to pain.

9. Back pain is an overtested and often overtreated problem (imaging, surgery, medication), due in part to the fact that many research studies have not been well-defined. Only about 1 percent of people with back pain require surgery. It is believed that there are almost twenty times more back operations per capita in the U.S. than Canada, and the fact is that this does not result in a greater treatment success rate. Surgery is definitely overdone.

In next section, we will first summarize those methods commonly used for diagnosis today, followed by a description of different popular Western treatments. Then, some suggestions from Western medicine for preventing back pain and some important tips for posture will be provided in section 4-3.

4-2. Western Medical Treatments

In this section, we will first discuss the techniques of diagnosis that are in use today. From this discussion, you may increase your understanding of how back pain can begin. After this, we will summarize the possible treatments which are used by modern physicians.

Physical Diagnosis

History. Generally, a patient's history could reveal most of the clues for a correct diagnosis. For example, if the pain worsens when the patient is sitting, the probable diagnosis is disc disease. If the patient is most uncomfortable while standing, the facet joints are implicated. If the pain is aggravated by walking, the cause is most likely spinal stenosis. And if the pain is worst when the patient is recumbent, a space-occupying lesion may possibly be the reason.

Physical Examinations. During acute pain, muscle spasm will lateralize to the side of the pathology, occasionally producing a pelvic tilt. The maintenance of lordosis at any point between L1 and S1 on flexion indicates a lack of motion and localizes the pathology.

Another cause of lower back pain is often unequal leg lengths. This can be measured from the anterior superior iliac spine to the medial malleous bilaterally.

Tests. A number of tests can assist the physician in making the diagnosis:

1. The straight-leg-raising test (SLR) for radiculopathy is positive when pain is produced between 30 and 60 degrees (When a patient's leg is raised less than 30 degrees, no stretch is produced; when it is raised more than 60 degrees, even mechanical pain can produce a positive result.) The SLR is useful for the L4-5 and L5-S1 discs only. Some 98 percent of herniated discs involve these two levels.

2. The femoral stretch test for disc disease at L2-4 is performed by flexing the knee while the patient is in the prone position with the hip extended. Older individuals have a higher risk of disc herniation at these upper lumbar levels.

3. The FABER test (for flexion, abduction, and external rotation of the hip) is useful for localizing the source of pain in the lumbar region if the hip and the S1 joint can be excluded.

Neurologic Examinations. Reflexes that have been lost during a previous episode of lumbar radiculopathy rarely return, even when there has been full motor recovery. The same is true for a finding of radiculopathy on electromyelography (EMG); once it is present, it may be permanent. This can lead to an over interpretation of the EMG on the physical exam during subsequent attacks of lower back pain. An experienced neurologist can usually distinguish acute changes from chronic ones on EMG.

Differential Diagnosis[4]

X-rays. Plain X-rays are not necessary to diagnose acute back pain unless the pain is associated with objective radiculopathy (i.e., disease of the spinal roots). The chance of finding any significant additional information is too small. Normally, X-rays are used only when the pain has lasted beyond a month.

But again, there are times when X-rays are necessary:

1. Trauma, of course, requires films to determine if there is any fracture, subluxation, or soft tissue mass.

2. Systemic Symptoms—for example, morning stiffness, weight loss, or fever— also necessitate X-rays.

3. X-rays are needed when there is the possibility of a *developmental or heritable* condition in a young person.

4. When facet arthritis is a consideration, oblique films should be included in the survey.

CAT Scans (computerized axial tomography). When back pain remains unexplained, a bone scan should be ordered. CAT scans are special X-rays used with a computer to produce images of a "slice" of anatomic tissue. They are good for looking at the spinal cord, spinal bones, fractures, osteoarthritis damage, narrowed spinal canal (spinal stenosis), tumors, and spinal cord infections.

Myelogram. A myelogram is another type of X-ray examination. Before taking X-rays, the radiologist injects a contrast medium (dye) into the spinal canal. This dye blocks X-rays and outlines the spinal cord and spinal nerves. Myelograms can show a ruptured disc.

MRI (magnetic resonance imaging). MRI uses a strong magnetic field and a computer to created highly detailed images of soft tissues, such as muscles, cartilage, ligaments, tendons, blood vessels and to a lesser extent, bone. MRI can also show disc degeneration, protrusion and rupture, infection and other spinal disorders.

EMG (electromyogram). EMG is a graphic record of muscle contraction that can show nerve and muscle damage.

Back Pain Treatments

In the last decade, a new concept of treatment has arisen and has been proven to work well, at least no worse than traditional methods. The trend is away from passive therapies and toward greater self-reliance and a return to activity as soon as feasible. A "wait and see" interval could turn into a period of deconditioning. The more patients can do on their own and the sooner they can do it, the greater the physical as well as psychological benefits.

Next, we would like to summarize the general treatments for back pain. In this summary, both conservative traditional methods and new techniques are included. Therefore, use your own judgment in selecting the method for your case. Remember, even today, we still cannot be sure which techniques are more effective than others. Naturally, you should also realize that the effectiveness of a treatment also depends on how the problem was started. The better you can pinpoint the problem from diagnosis, the easier you may solve the problem.

Before we summarize the treatments, there are a few initial suggestions from Western medicine to consider if you are stricken with back pain:

1. Wait for the discomfort to calm down before you begin to stimulate or actively move your back muscles.

2. Once you feel more comfortable, stay active if you can and if possible, resume physical activity as soon as possible.

3. If the pain is extreme, use medications wisely and cautiously. Avoid narcotics if at all possible.

4. If you so desire, see a chiropractor once or twice. It may be a simple spinal alignment problem which causes tension in the muscles on the back. Sometimes, a chiropractor is able to correct the problem in a short time.

5. The last method is seeing a doctor and undergoing a physical. Most patients don't need X-rays. Often a few simple questions will identify those who do.

General Treatments of Back Pain[1 & 5]

Short Period of Rest. The most basic treatment for acute back pain is a short period of rest, no more than two days. In the past, one to two weeks of bed rest was recommended by physicians. However, a recent study has reported that resting longer than two days is not necessarily more effective than only two days of bed rest.[6 & 7] Moreover, there is no firm scientific evidence to show that bed rest is beneficial, nevertheless there is ample evidence of the deleterious effects of bed rest. In fact, there is a 3 percent loss of muscle strength per day during bed rest, resulting in decreased physical fitness. Prolonged rest can only lead to depression, loss of working habits, and difficulty in starting rehabilitation.

So far, there is no indication that activity is harmful or makes the pain worse in the long-term. On the contrary, increased activity promises to promote bone and muscle strength, and may also increase endorphin levels. People who keep physically fit are at less risk for episodes of back pain. Activity is not harmful, and active rehabilitation helps to restore function and reduce pain.

Applications of Ice or Heat. Applications of ice or heat to the aching area is probably one of the most common treatments for any pain. In ice therapy, ice packs or ice massage is applied or rubbed over the painful area for fifteen minutes every hour or more; this can alleviate acute pain. If ice is applied, a towel should be placed over the skin to protect it.

Moist heat is an alternative to ice therapy. When heat is used, the patient can be more relaxed and feel comfortable, and the blood circulation can be improved. Consequently, pain and stiffness can be eased. In heat therapy, moist warm towels can be used by themselves or in combination with a heating pad. In order to avoid burns and the generation of negative effects, heating pads should not be left on for more than thirty minutes.

Medications.[4] Often, medications are used to ease pain or reduce discomfort. However, you must recognize two important facts. First, medications can only solve the symptoms temporarily, but not the root. Once the effectiveness of the medication ends, the discomfort will normally return. Second, almost all medications generate side-effects. Therefore, if you decide to take medications, you should consider all of these factors.

For non-prescription medicine, **acetaminophen** and **ibuprofen** can help relieve pain and swelling. There are also many medications which can help reduce discomfort. **Narcotic analgesics** can decrease discomfort. However, narcotics can cause constipation and depression, decrease function, and suppress natural endorphins.

One of the most common types of medication ordered are muscle relaxants, such as **cyclobenzaprine (Flexeril)**, **methocarbamol (Robaxin)**, or **carisoprodol (Soma)**. There is little evidence to support their efficacy. The most common side effect of muscle relaxants is drowsiness.

Frequently nonsteroidal anti-inflammatory medications (**NSAIDs**) are prescribed. These medications block prostaglandin production and reduce inflammation, thus helping the pain. There are many side effects of their usage, including gastro-intestinal distress, such as nausea, heartburn, and diarrhea; kidney impairment; and fluid retention. No one group of NSAIDs has proven more effective than any other group.[7] Failure with one NSAID should not deter trying others. Short-term systemic corticosteroids are still occasionally prescribed, but it should be stressed that even short-term use may cause significant long-term side effects.

Physical Therapy Modalities. Physical therapy using **TENS units (transcutaneous electrical nerve stimulation), diathermy, ultrasonagraphy, and hydrotherapy** may be prescribed. They may reduce muscle spasms and pain temporarily. When used in combination with exercise, these methods may facilitate earlier mobilization and improve function. Controlled studies have yet to show the effectiveness of these modalities alone. In fact, a study at the Seattle Veterans Affairs Medical Center shows that the effectiveness of reducing the pain from stretching exercises is as good as or better than the results generated by TENS.

Exercises. Today, **experts estimate that between 70 percent to 90 percent of back pain is caused by muscle or ligament problems, usually related to weakness in the lower back, rather than by serious damage to the spine itself.** From their experience, it is believed that most of the problems can be cleared up within a few weeks. However, if the strength of the lower back is not built up to a healthy level, most likely the pain will return. It is common that most doctors treat the pain, not the underlying disorder that caused the pain. Consequently, when patients go back to their unchanged life style, they end up hurting themselves again.[2]

Since the late 1980's many Western medical scientists have hypothesized that the best cure for back pain and the prevention of relapse is to strengthen the back muscles through exercise. That means muscular rehabilitation. This new concept of treatment is to emphasize not only treating the pain, but also to keep the patient up and about as much as possible to avoid the debilitation that results from inactivity. Routine use of medications and invasive modalities is discouraged. Naturally, this is a revolutionary concept which differs from the traditional Western medical suggestion which advised that the patient take medicine and then rest. Back treatment programs are now changing from **traditional rest and drug therapy to a new approach of aggressive exercise.**[1]

A variety of exercise programs have been developed to treat back pain, and the results have been significant. Some experts found that isometric exercises are the most effective.[8] Exercise should be started gradually and gently at first, increasing as the recovery process continues. Daily activities should also be encouraged, increased activity will promote bone and muscle strength and also increase endorphin levels. In fact, there is no evidence that early return to work will increase the future recurrence of back pain. Patients should be urged to gradually increase their fitness levels. According to one report, it was discovered that those in the most physically fit group were ten times less likely to develop back aches than those in the least physically fit group.

Corset or Brace. Corsets and braces decrease motion in the lumbar spine but do not achieve complete immobilization. It has been found that there is more relief of back pain by a corset with spinal support than by one without such support.[9]

Corsets increase intraabdominal pressure and may decrease intradiscal pressure.[3] The primary disadvantage of brace usage is a loss of muscle function leading to local muscle weakness. An exercise program to maintain muscle function should therefore accompany brace usage.

Manipulation. The most controversial treatment for back pain is spinal manipulation. No clear-cut guidelines or indications exist for the use of manipulation. There is no clear understanding for how manipulation works. Manipulations are expected to increase mobility, readjust the vertebrae, reduce the size of disc herniations, reduce spasms, and most of all decrease pain. Short-term manipulation by chiropractors or osteopaths may temporarily decrease pain and improve function.[10] But when the problem is disc herniation or osteoporosis, manipulation may make matters worse.

Back School. One of the most important aspects of back pain treatment is education. It has been recognized that education is the most effective form of back pain treatment.[11] Back school is a program that provides in-depth information about anatomy of the spine, exercises, and body mechanics to help individuals with back pain manage their symptoms and minimize future injury. This can best be done by a nurse or physician who understands the mechanisms of back pain and its medical management. Patients with back pain often have difficulty dealing with the pain, becoming discouraged by its effect on their daily lives and quality of living, and experiencing frustration with the medical community's inability to provide a cure. Through educational programs, patients can understand their condition and build up confidence in dealing with the problem both physically and psychologically.

Surgery.[4] It was estimated in 1987 that fewer than 10 percent of the cases of lower back pain required surgery. Moreover, out of the surgeries performed, only about 75 percent really got great results. It is believed that often the wrong operation is done or an operation is done on a patient who could have gotten by without one.

Although physicians prefer to treat even severe cases of lower back pain in a conservative manner with bed rest and painkillers, surgery is clearly called for if pressure on a nerve root causes severe pain lasting for weeks, or if progressive damage to the nerves results in leg weakness or paralysis. Every year, about twenty thousand Americans undergo surgery for persistent back pain.

The most common surgery is the removal of the slipped or herniated disc. In this operation, the doctors get at the disc by removing only a very small part of the bone—the arch of the vertebra (this procedure is called a laminectomy). Then, they remove the part of the disc that is out of place and any other loose fragments that are accessible.

Another condition that requires laminectomy is spinal stenosis, an unusual narrowing of the space inside the spinal canal. A narrow spinal canal may cause pressure on the nerve roots and, in rare cases, on the cord itself. This is the second most common operation for back pain treatment. The reason for this necessity is that some people are born with a narrow spinal canal, while some others develop a buildup of ligaments and bone spurs that also narrow the spinal canal. This results in wear and tear, and having the spine work against gravity over time.

In some cases, spinal fusion is done. Because the spine is made up of a number of joints, and if a joint is unstable and slips, causing nerve root pinching, the slipping is stopped by fusing the two vertebrae together. To do this, surgeons insert fragments of the patient's own bone, usually taken from the hip, to bridge the space between two adjacent vertebrae. In time, the bones grow together. Fusion relieves pain but reduces mobility.

Other Treatments.[4] In a small percentage of cases, sciatic pain caused by a herniated disc that would normally required surgery is treated by some physicians with chymopapain. This drug, approved by the FDA in 1982, is an enzyme found in papaya that is used to tenderize meat, make beer, and clear cloudy contact lenses. Injected into the disc's jelly-like center, chymopapain dissolves the disc, thus lessening pressure on the nerve root. The drug has had its champions and detractors ever since it was introduced, but when used in patients in whom conservative treatment has failed and who are candidates for surgery, it can be very successful. Its advantages over surgery are a shorter hospital stay, less expense, less scarring and less trauma. Since some people are highly allergic to the drug, skin tests must be done first to detect chymopapain sensitivity in candidates for treatment.

A relatively new technique called **aspiration percutaneous lumbar discectomy (APLD)** may be useful for people allergic to chymopapain and those for whom general anesthesia is risky. Using X-ray pictures as a guide, the neurosurgeon or orthopedist inserts a long, thin needle called a nucleotome probe into the center of the protruding disc. The physician loosens the disc material by moving the probe back and force. A pump that is attached to the probe suctions up the material and carries it away.

APLD takes about forty minutes, requires about ten days recuperation, and costs a great deal less than laminectomy. However, not everybody is a suitable candidate for this procedure. It cannot be used on those who have severely ruptured discs or spinal stenosis.

4-3. Suggestions from Western Doctors

In our early education, we become attached to the notion that pain means sickness. We do not recognize that pain is a signal from the body to inform the mind that we are doing something wrong, not necessarily that something is wrong. Often, instead of addressing ourselves to the cause, we turn to pills, driving the pain underground. Consequently, sickness is generated and the condition continues to worsen. According to Chinese medicine and Qigong, pain or any feeling of discomfort is actually the language that the body uses to communicate with the brain. If the brain does not register this message, serious and chronic problems will eventually manifest. One of the most important parts of Chinese Qigong is learning how to feel the body's condition. This kind of training is called "internal vision" (i.e., internal feeling).

In this section, we will summarize a number of valuable suggestions and tips from Western doctors for back pain prevention. These suggestions will not only help you correct the possibly already wrong life style which you may have for future back pain, but also provide you with a better awareness of and alertness to your body's signals or condition. Only when you have this awareness can you appreciate the early warning signs of a problem and prevent it from getting worse.

Suggestions:[1]

Education. The most important method of preventing the occurrence of back pain is education. First, you should understand the anatomic structure of your back, especially the spine. Next, you must research the possible causes of back pain. Naturally, reading or studying other patients' experiences can always bring attention and awareness to your own situation.

If possible, try to understand the existing treatments. Since it is almost impossible to pinpoint the cause of back pain and the treatment effectiveness is often vague, it might be **wise to examine and use both the Western and Eastern methods of treatment**. Finally, you should study your life style and analyze your body's condition both physically and mentally. Only through these educational processes can you direct yourself to a healthy life path.

Use Common Sense. Before you can apply your common sense to an action, you must first build up a habit of awareness and alertness. Once you can bring yourself to attention, then you can analyze the situation and make a wise judgment. For example, do you use a bad sitting posture while watching television? If you can bring awareness and thought to it, you can correct this mistake before any problem starts. Other examples are, do you use safe lifting and handling techniques and body mechanics? Does your workplace make you feel depressed or tense? Naturally, the more you are educated about the spine's structure and possible pain causes, the better you can correct any problems. The key is to be aware of the body's condition and the activities involved. When you use your common sense to make judgments, you can avoid most injuries or problems.

Later, we will list a few keys to spine protection from different situations and body postures.

Stay Physically Fit. The next important means to prevent back pain from occurring is to keep your body in a physically healthy condition. This includes the compact bone structure, as well as the strength of the ligaments, tendons and muscles. When these factors are strong, you will have a firm and solid foundation to keep your physical body in a balanced condition. When your body is in a balanced state, the torso posture will be correct, and the strains and stresses on the spine will be minimized.

The best way to keep this balance is to improve the strength of the back's extensor muscles, which allow you to uncurl from a tucked position and stand upright against gravity. When the extensors are weak, the pelvis tips forward, robbing the lower back of support, and the hamstring and hip muscles end up taking over most of the lower back's load. This creates tightness in the hamstrings and hips, and leaves the lower back chronically weak.[2]

Therefore, correct ways of exercising to maintain the health of the muscles and spine are important. With the correct exercises, those muscles that support the spine and reduce its strain will be strengthened. Wrong exercises may either cause back pain or worsen it. Moreover, you must also know that **exercise and relaxation should mutually balance each other**. Too much exercise can make your muscles fatigued and more strained or tightened. Too much resting will make the muscles degenerate and weaken.

In fact, the hardest part of maintaining physical strength is not learning exercises, but maintaining an exercise schedule. Often, we are easily conquered by our lazy mind and quit. Truly, it is our mind that makes our bodies both physically and mentally weak and degenerate. Therefore, the keys to preventing yourself from getting sick are learning to conquer yourself and establishing a healthy life style.

Stress Reduction. It is well known that emotional strain can cause back muscles to tighten and therefore increase the stress on the spinal joints. Often, mental stress originates from an abnormal life style, from mental anxiety, from an unhappy job environment or from feelings of guilt. If this is the case, then you must first analyze and learn the cause of your stress and correct it. If this cause is not corrected, the problem will return.

In Western medicine, one of the possible treatments for tightened back muscles is to make the patient exercise in a pool while wearing a buoyant vest with weights suspended from the waist. The idea is to stretch the spine and attached muscles. This treatment has been reported to result in an 80 percent to 85 percent improvement among patients.[5]

Some machines such as the MedX back and neck machine developed by Arthur Jones, inventor of the Nautilus weight machine, are able to hold the patient's pelvis down tight with restraining mechanisms controlled by a therapist. Once the lower body is immobilized, the patient, who is sitting in a tucked position, pushes backward with the upper body against preset resistance, working just the lower back muscles.

Avoid or Stop Smoking. According to statistical analysis, it is believed that there is a possible relationship between symptomatic disc disease, such as prolapsed lumbar disc and a prolapsed cervical disc of the spine, and cigarette smoking.[12] The fact is that most patients with symptomatic disc disease and a majority of the patients with acute lumbar disc herniation who undergo surgery are smokers. Theoretically, it is possible that smoking is related to decreased blood oxygenation to the disc, which interferes with the repair process of the body, specifically the disc, and thus it ages or degenerates prematurely. Smokers also cough more than nonsmokers, which increases the pounds of pressure on the disc, resulting in increased physical stress to the disc. Naturally, in order to quit your smoking habit, you must first conquer yourself mentally.

Avoid Obesity. To maintain your normal weight is one of the keys to insure that the trunk will not carry any additional physical load. Moreover, because of greater abdominal girth, a obese individual normally is a greater distance from the objects he or she is lifting. Furthermore, he or she may also have more difficulty squatting to lift. The fact is that the farther away an object is from the individual's center of gravity, the higher the risk for strain to the lower back.

Important Tips on Body Posture

Sitting:

1. Avoid sitting in one place or in one position for a long time. Get up and stretch, walk about, and change positions. Bring your awareness and common sense into your consciousness. Often, placing a cushion or rolled-up towel under your back can help you feel more comfortable.

2. If you sit for a long time, rest your feet on a low stool. But do not generate more tension in the knee area which may cause injury to the knees. Keep your knees bent.

3. Avoid sitting in soft, deep seats. If you are having back pain, try to sit in a chair with arms that will help you get up and down.

4. At a desk or in the car, sit so your knees are level with your hips. This will reduce some of the stress on the lower back.

5. When driving, adjust the seat so your legs don't have to stretch to reach the pedals. In addition, you should get out and stretch every twenty to thirty minutes. This will loosen your torso and reduce the strain on the lower back.

Lifting:[1]

1. Think before moving. Again, this is an awareness of the conditions around you and use of your common sense to make a wise judgment.

2. Clear the area of clutter. Before you lift, you should check around you and clear the space. This will give you a better maneuvering area if you have problems lifting.

3. Test the load. Before you lift, test it first. This will help you understand your capability and the potential for injury.

4. Keep all lifted objects close to your body. When you lift, the closer the object is to you, the better balance you will have and therefore, the less strain you will have on your back muscles.

5. Use a wide, balanced stance like a weight lifter. In order to have good balance when you lift, you should keep your legs apart and seek for the best balance and most comfortable position.

6. Avoid lifting anything while you are reaching, twisting or bending forward. Also, you should avoid jerking while lifting.

7. When lifting, bend your knees and use the force of your legs to help lift in a smooth motion. Don't bend over at the waist with your legs straight.

8. Tighten the back and abdominal muscles. This will protect your ligaments and vertebrae and help prevent injury.

9. Don't lift a heavy load above your waist. It will definitely be worse if the height is above your chest.

10. Avoid lifting more than 35 percent of your body weight without help.

11. Use lumbar belts. Lumbar belts are used to prevent back muscle injuries by prohibiting poor lifting techniques and employing other muscles to perform the majority of the work. Be aware though that, according to one study, belts do not increase the strength of the lower back muscles or help the wearer lift heavier weights.

Sleeping:

1. Use a firm mattress. Too soft or too rigid is not good for the back.

2. Find a sleeping position that is most comfortable. This may mean sleeping on your side with your knees bent, on your back or side with a pillow under your knees or not using a pillow at all.

3. Never sleep on your stomach. Sleeping on your stomach will not help your back pain problems. Sleeping this way will normally exaggerate your pain, and often creates neck pain and headaches.

Walking:

1. Try to take a brisk walk every day. Be sure to wear comfortable, well-cushioned low heeled shoes.

2. Wear comfortable, appropriate clothing. Tight clothes make you feel uneasy, especially in the torso. Loose and comfortable clothes can make you relax and feel free when you walk.

References

1. "Outpatient Management of Lower Back Pain," Judith A. Chase, *Orthopedic Nursing,* January/February 1992, Vol. 11/No. 1.

2. *The Back Power Program*, Dr. David Imrie, John Wiley and Sons, 1990.

3. "Back Pain and Sciatica," Frymoyer, J., *New England Journal of Medicine,* 318(5), 1988, 291-300.

4. *Back Talk: Advice for Suffering Spines*, Evelyn Zamula, FDA Consumer, April 1989.

5. "Backaches," Oliver Fultz, *American Health,* November 1991.

6. "Office Management of Lower Back Pain," Lee, C., *Orthopedic Clinics of North America,* 19(4), 797-804, 1988.

7. "Low Back Disorders: Conservative Management," Fast, A., *Archives of Physical Medicine and Rehabilitation,* 69(10), 880-891, 1988.

8. "A Randomized Controlled Trial of Flexion Exercises, Education, and Bed Rest for Patients with Acute lower Back Pain," Evans, C., Gilbert, J., Taylor, W., et al., *Physiotherapy Canada,* 39(2), 1987, 96-101.

9. "Assessment of the Progress of the Back-Pain Patient," Million, R., Hall, W., Nilsen, K., et al., *Spine,* 7(3), 1987, 204-212.

10. "Conservative Therapy for Lower Back Pain," Deyo, R., *Journal of American Medical Association,* 250(8), 1983, 1057-1062.

11. "Rationalized Approach to Physiotherapy for the Back Pain," Sikorski, J., *Spine,* 10(6), 1985.

12. "Studies Find Adverse Affects of Cigarette Smoking," Alvin Nagelberg and Joanne Swanson, *P. M. Release,* Thursday, Feb. 18, 1993, Paper 8 and 520.

13. "Acute and Chronic Low Back Pain: How to Pinpoint its Cause and Make the Diagnosis," Burton Sack, M.D., *Modern Medicine,* 58, September, 1992.

CHAPTER 5

How do the Chinese Treat Back Pain?

中醫治背疼的方法

5-1. Introduction

In the first chapter, we said that the definition of Qigong is "the study of Qi." This means that Qigong actually covers a very wide field of research, and includes the study of the three general types of Qi (Heaven Qi, Earth Qi, and Human Qi) and their interrelationships. However, because the Chinese have traditionally paid more attention to the study of Human Qi, which is concerned with health and longevity, the term "Qigong" has often been misunderstood and misused to mean only the study of Human Qi. Because so much attention has been given to Human Qi over thousands of years, human Qigong has reached a very high level. Today it includes many fields such as acupuncture, herbal study, massage, cavity press, Qigong exercises, martial arts, and even spiritual enlightenment.

In this chapter, I would like to summarize, according to my understanding, some of the methods commonly used in China to prevent back pain and to cure it. I would then like to focus the discussion on how Qigong uses exercises and massage (including cavity press) to prevent and cure back pain.

5-2. General Chinese Treatments for Back Pain

Since Chinese diagnosis is not quite as familiar to the general Western public, in this section, we will first summarize the general diagnostic techniques of Chinese medicine. Then, a special diagnosis for back pain will be reviewed. After this, general treatments for back pain in Chinese medicine will be discussed.

Chinese Medical Diagnosis

person is sick, his Qi circulation is irregular or abnormal—it is too Yin or
ecause all Qi channels are connected to the surface of the body, stagnant
or abnormal Qi flow will cause signs to show on the skin. Also, the sounds a sick person makes when speaking, coughing, or breathing are different from those of a healthy person. Chinese doctors therefore examine a patient's skin, particularly the forehead, eyes, ears, and tongue. They also pay close attention to the person's sounds. In addition, they ask the patient a number of questions about his daily habits, hobbies, and feelings to understand the background of the illness. Finally, the doctor feels the pulses and probes special spots on the body to further check the condition of specific channels. Therefore, Chinese diagnosis is divided into four principal categories: 1. Looking (Wang Zhen, 望診); 2. Listening and Smelling (Wen Zhen, 聞診); 3. Asking (Wen Zhen, 問診); and 4. Palpation (Qie Zhen, 切診).

Obviously Chinese medicine takes a somewhat different approach to diagnosis than Western medicine does. Chinese doctors treat the body as a whole, analyzing the cause of the illness from the patient's appearance and behavior. Often what the Chinese physician considers important clues or causes are viewed by the Western doctor as symptomatic or irrelevant, and vice versa.

Next, we will briefly discuss the above four Chinese diagnostic techniques:

Looking (Wang Zhen, 望診):

Looking at the spirit and inspecting the color:

1. General Appearance: Examine the facial expression, muscle tone, posture, and general spirit.

2. Skin Color: Examine the skin color of the injured area, if the problem is externally visible, like a bruise or pulled muscle. Examine the skin color of the face (Figure 5-1). Since some channels are connected to the face, its color can tell the Chinese doctor what organs are disordered or out of balance.

3. Tongue: The tongue is closely connected through channels with the heart, kidney, stomach, liver, gall bladder, lungs, and spleen (Figure 5-2). In making his diagnosis, the Chinese doctor will check the shape, fur, color, and the body of the tongue to determine the condition of the organs.

4. Eyes: From the appearance of the eyes a doctor can tell the liver condition. For example, when the eyes are red, it means the liver has too much Yang. Also, black spots on the whites of the eyes (Figure 5-3), can tell of problems with the Qi circulation, degeneration of organs, or stagnancy due to an old injury.

5. Hair: The condition of the hair can indicate the health of the kidneys and the blood. For example, thin, dry hair indicates deficient kidney Qi or weak blood.

6. Lip and Gums: The color of the lips and their relative dryness indicates if the Qi is deficient or exhausted. Red, swollen, or bleeding gums can be caused by

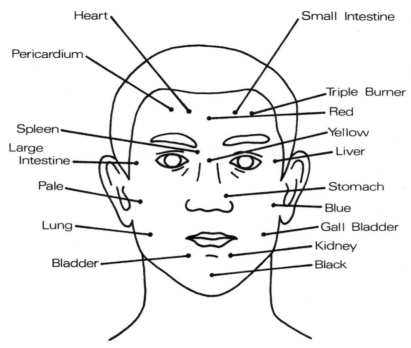

Figure 5-1. Diagnosis from the Face's Color

stomach fire. Pale, swollen gums and loose teeth might be a symptom of deficient kidneys.

Listening and Smelling
(Wen Zhen, 聞診):

1. Listening to patient's breathing, mode of speech and cough. For example, a dry, hacking cough is caused by dry heat in the lungs.

2. Smelling the odor of a patient's breath and excrement. For example, in the case of diseases caused by excessive heat, the various secretions and excretions of the body have a heavy, foul odor, while in diseases caused by excessive cold, they smell more like rotten fish.

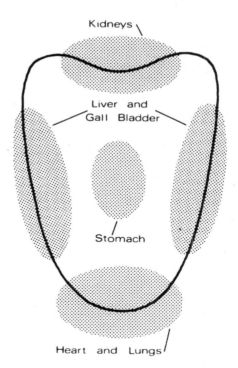

Figure 5-2. Diagnosis from the Tongue's Condition

127

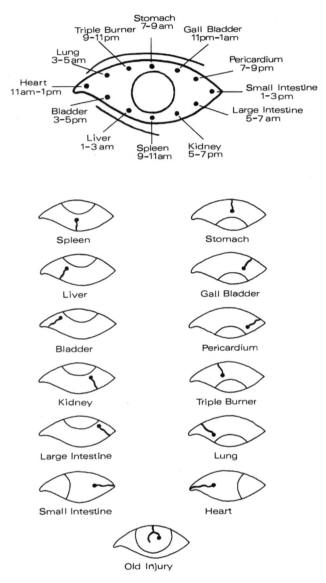

Figure 5-3. Diagnosis from the Eyes' Black (or Blue) Spots and Lines

Asking (Wen Zhen, 問診):

This is one of the most important sources of a successful diagnosis. The questions usually cover the patient's past medical history, present condition, habits and life style. Traditionally, there are ten main subjects a Chinese doctor will focus on in this interview. They are:

1. Chills and fever
2. Head and body

3. Perspiration
4. Diet and appetite
5. Urine and stool
6. Chest and abdomen
7. Eyes and ears
8. Sleep
9. Medical history
10. Bearing and living habits

Palpation (Qie Zhen, 切診):

There are three major forms of palpation (touching or feeling) in Chinese medicine:

1. The palpation of areas which feel painful, hot, swollen, etc. to determine the nature of the problem. For example, swelling and heat indicates there is too much Yang in the area.

2. The palpation of specific acupuncture points on the front and back of the trunk. For example, if the doctor senses a collapsed feeling, or the point is sore to touch, this indicates the possibility of disease in the organ with which the point is associated.

3. The palpation of pulse: Traditionally, the radial area pulse on the wrist (Figure 5-4) is the principal site for pulse diagnosis. Although the pulse is specially related to the lungs and controlled by the heart, it refers the condition of all

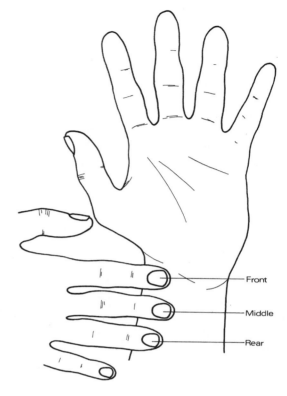

Figure 5-4. The Palpation of the Pulse

Table 5-1
The Palpatation of the Pulse

Left Hand	Organs
Rear	Kidney Yin
Middle	Liver
Front	Heart

Right Hand	Organs
Rear	Kidney Yang
Middle	Spleen
Front	Lungs

organs (Table 5-1). The doctor checks the following: the depth (floating or submerged), the pace (slow or fast), the length (long or short), the strength (weak or strong), and the quality (slippery, rough, wiry, tight, huge, fine, or irregular). Usually it takes several years and hundreds of cases to become expert in the palpation of pulse.

Recently, inspection of skin eruptions on the ears has been used in Chinese diagnosis. A number of sites have been found on the ear which become spontaneously tender or otherwise react to disease or injury somewhere in the body. Stimulation of these ear points in turn exerts certain therapeutic effects on those parts of the body with which they are associated. Moreover, many Western diagnostic methods, such as using X-rays, have also been adopted to coordinate with Chinese diagnosis.

This section serves only as a brief introduction to Chinese medical diagnosis. Interested readers should refer to books about Chinese medicine for more information.

Next, we will list the possible diagnostic techniques for back pain. However, before we begin, first let us see how the Chinese define back pain or pain associated with back. The most common term for back pain is called Yaotong (腰痛 , lumbago)—waist pain. From this, you can see most back pain is in the waist area (i.e., lumbar vertebrae). It is also called Yaokaotong (腰尻痛 , lumbosacral pain)—pain in the lumbar vertebrae. However, when the pain has reached to the upper section of the spine, it is called Yaojitong (腰脊痛)—pain along the spinal column. If the pain in the waist area is only sore without severe pain, it is called Yaosuan (腰酸)—soreness of waist. And if the entire back is aching it is called Yaobeitengtong (腰背疼痛)—pain in the back and loins, lumbago and back pain.

From this terminology you can see that according to Chinese medical definitions, back pain is not a disease, but the pain is caused from some special sickness. Therefore, the beginning treatment is to stop the pain and then follow with some herbal treatments or special Qigong exercises to heal the sickness or to rebuild the strength of the physical and/or Qi bodies. It is believed that only then will the root of the sickness be removed, and further sickness prevented.

Diagnosis for Back Pain

1. Looking and inspecting the postures of the patient to see if there is any abnormal structure in or appearance of the spine.
2. Asking the patient and understanding the patient's medical history and conditions. Where is the pain? How did the back pain start? How long have the symptoms existed? When is the pain most severe?
3. Palpating the areas which feel painful, hot, swollen, etc. to determine the nature of the problem. Also, from the hands' touch on special areas or cavities on the back, an experienced Chinese physician is able to tell where the Qi is stagnant in the back.
4. From different angles of arm or leg movement, or different angles of the torso's gentle twisting and bending, some special injuries or muscular spasms can be identified.

General Chinese Treatments for Back Pain

As mentioned earlier, back pain is not considered to be a sickness, but a pain caused from other sicknesses. Therefore, the usual treatment is first to stop the pain by using either acupuncture and/or massage. The key to reaching this goal is to improve the Qi and blood circulation in the pained area. Occasionally, herbs are also used to improve the circulation and stop the pain. However, all of these efforts are considered temporary, since they are not able to cure the root of the sickness but only alleviate the symptoms. In order to have a complete recovery or to cure the root of the problem, a healthy and strong foundation must be rebuilt. Naturally, this usually takes a long time, but it is a long term solution.

Therefore, a Chinese physician will treat the painful symptoms and try to make the patient more comfortable, and he will teach the patient some special Qigong breathing techniques and movements to either expedite the recovery from sickness or to rebuild the strength of the body.

As matter of fact, the best way to maintain health is to prevent sickness from occurring. It is the same for back pain. The best way to prevent it from occurring is to be aware of your life style and to keep your body in good condition. However, if it has already occurred, then the appropriate course is to prevent it from getting any worse, and learn to rebuild the physical strength of the back so that it can resume functioning normally.

In this section, we will briefly discuss the theory of several common methods for treating back pain which have been developed in China. The actual treating techniques will be discussed in the next chapter.

Massage. When done properly, massage will improve the Qi and blood circulation in the joint areas. Improved circulation can ease pain and help the patient feel more comfortable.

Generally speaking, Chinese massage can be classified into four categories according to their purposes. They are:

1. **General Massage (Pu Tong An Mo, 普通按摩).** General massage is the most common and popular massage. The purposes of general massage are simple and the techniques are relatively easier than the other three categories. The main goals of this massage are: a. relaxation; b. recovery from fatigue; c. preventing illness; d. slowing down aging; e. speeding recovery from sudden environmental Qi disturbance; and f. enjoyment.

   From these, you can see that general massage is not aiming for healing, but for improving the Qi and blood circulation for different purposes. Normally, a Chinese masseur will start his or her training from general massage. This is simply because through general massage practice, you can master the basic massage techniques and also get a better acquaintance with human anatomy and the Qi status of the body.

2. **Push Grab Massage (Tui Na An Mo, 推拿按摩).** Tui Na massage is often simply called Tui Na. Tui Na means "push" and "grab," and refers to the two major techniques. Tui Na has two main purposes: a. treating injuries; and b. treating illnesses, especially in small children. When Tui Na is used for treating injuries, the main goal is to remove any blood stagnation (i.e., bruises) and Qi blockage, thereby expediting the healing process. When it is used for

treating sickness, the main goal is to regulate the abnormal Qi circulation of the internal organs to a healthy state.

3. **Cavity Press Massage (Dian Xue An Mo, 點穴按摩).** Cavity Press (Dian Xue, 點穴) is the method of using the fingertips (especially the thumb tip) to press acupuncture cavities and certain other points (pressure points) on the body in order to manipulate the Qi circulation. Acupuncture cavities are tiny spots distributed over the entire body where the Qi of the body can be manipulated through massage or the insertion of needles. According to the new theory of bioelectricity, these cavities are places where the electrical conductivity is higher than in neighboring areas. They are therefore more sensitive to external stimulation, and allow this stimulation to reach to the primary Qi channels.[1]

The theory of cavity press is very similar to that of acupuncture. There are a few differences, however: a. acupuncture uses needles or other means of penetration such as lasers, while cavity press uses the fingertips to press the cavities; b. acupuncture can reach much deeper than cavity press; c. cavity press is easier and more convenient than acupuncture, which requires equipment and a higher level of training. This means that anyone can learn to use cavity press to treat back pain after only a short period of training and some experience. However, it takes years of study to learn acupuncture; d. a patient can use cavity press on himself or herself much more easily than acupuncture.

In cavity press, stagnant Qi deep in the joint can be led to the surface. This improves the Qi circulation in the joint area, and reduces pain considerably. The use of cavity press to speed up the healing of injured joints is very common in the Chinese martial arts.

4. **Qi Massage (Qi An Mo, 氣按摩).** Qi massage is commonly called "Wai Qi Liao Fa" (外氣療法), which means "curing with external Qi," and is commonly translated "Qi healing" in the West today. This term implies that the massage is done through Qi correspondence rather than touch.

To understand Qi massage, you must recognize that Qi is the bioelectricity circulating in the body. Because it is electricity, it can be conducted or led through electrical correspondence. Actually, everybody has the ability to do Qi healing. For example, when your friend is sad, her Qi status is Yin (i.e., deficient). If you hold her hands or hug her, your Qi will nourish her and she will immediately feel better. Humans have been doing this instinctively for a long time. The only difference between the average person and a Qigong master is that the latter has trained in Qi healing, and can therefore be more effective.

In Qi massage, a patient's back pain can be alleviated when the accumulated or stagnant Qi is led away from the painful area. This will make the patient more relaxed and feel more comfortable. Naturally, like other massage, the healing process can be expedited. If you are interested in knowing more about Chinese massage, please refer to the book *Chinese Qigong Massage*, from YMAA Publication Center.

Acupuncture. Acupuncture is another common method of temporarily stopping the pain and increasing the Qi circulation in the joint area to help the healing. The main difference between massage and acupuncture is that the former usually stays only on the surface, while the latter can reach to the center of the joint. One of the advantages of acupuncture is that, if the back pain is caused by an old injury deep in the joint, it can heal the injury or at least remove some of the stagnated Qi or bruising.

In acupuncture, needles or other newly developed means such as lasers or electricity are used to stimulate and increase the Qi circulation. Although acupuncture can stop the pain and can, to some degree, cure back pain, the process can be so time-consuming as to be emotionally draining. Acupuncture is an external method, and while it may remove the symptoms, it can usually heal back pain only temporarily or only to a limited degree. Rebuilding the strength of the joints in the spine is a long term proposition. Therefore, after back pain patients have received some treatment, the physician will frequently encourage them to get involved in Qigong exercises to rebuild the joints.

Herbal Treatments. Herbal treatments are used together with massage and acupuncture, especially when back pain is caused by an injury. The herbs are usually made into a plaster or ground into powder, mixed with a liquid such as alcohol, and then applied to the joint. The dressing is changed every twenty-four hours.

Herbal treatments are used to alleviate pain, to increase the Qi circulation and help the healing of injury, and to speed up the process of re-growth. Often oral herbs are prescribed by a Chinese physician to stop the pain and also to expedite the healing process.

Qigong Exercises. The main purpose of Qigong exercise for back pain is to rebuild the strength of the joint by improving the Qi circulation. As mentioned earlier, traditional Chinese physicians believe that since the body's cells are alive, as long as there is a proper supply of Qi, physical damage can be repaired or even completely rebuilt. They have proven that broken bones can be mended completely, even in the elderly. Even some Western physicians have now come to believe that damaged or degenerated joints can re-grow to their original healthy state.[2]

Let us now summarize the similarities and differences in how Chinese and Western medicine treat back pain.

Summary:

Diagnosis

1. Neither Western nor Chinese diagnosis can pinpoint the cause of back pain clearly.

2. Western diagnosis is more detailed, and disease or injury is diagnosed upon the theory that seeing is believing. Therefore, all diagnoses originate from an anatomical point of view. Different high-tech instruments have been developed to view internal physical problems. However, although Chinese medicine today also uses X-rays for diagnosis, traditionally the diagnosis depended on surface appearance and feeling.

3. In Western diagnosis, different terminology has been created to explain the possible causes of back pain. There are not many different terms in Chinese medicine for back pain. In Chinese medicine, normally the causes of back pain are identified as only: muscular/tendon spasm, Qi stagnation, bone fracture, ligament injury, and/or arthritis. From this, you can see that it is much clearer to identify different causes of back pain from a Western point of view.

Treatments

1. Both Western and Chinese medicine use massage to alleviate pain by improving Qi and blood circulation.

2. Western medicine uses both ice and heat to ease pain and inflammation, while Chinese medicine uses only heat. This is because Chinese doctors believe that the ice treatment can only slow down the Qi and blood circulation and make the Qi and blood condense deeper into the joint, thus hindering the healing process.

3. Western medicine uses drugs to make the body relax and to ease pain. However, side effects have been widely noticed. Chinese medicine often uses acupuncture and external herbal treatments to ease pain, keep swelling down, and to improve Qi and blood circulation. Occasionally, internal herbs are used to keep swelling down, remove bruises, prevent further infection of the joints, and to expedite the healing by improving Qi and blood circulation. Normally, there are no or very minimal side effects from Chinese herbal treatments.

4. Western medicine teaches patients physical exercises to strengthen and rebuild the spine. However, Chinese Qigong teaches patients how to use the mind, coordinated with the correct breathing techniques, to enhance the Qi storage and circulation internally while also using physical Qigong movements to rebuild the strength and health of the vertebrae. A more detailed discussion of the differences in using Western physical exercise and Chinese Qigong for spinal rejuvenation will be included in the next section.

5. Western medicine is not concerned with the Qi status when a patient has a back pain problem. However, Chinese medicine pays great attention to it. Teaching a patient how to rebuild the Qi level and enhance the Qi circulation in the injured area is considered an important key to the healing process.

Prevention

In Western medicine and health care, there are few documents which discuss how to prevent back pain from occurring. Only in the last two decades has there been much information available on the factors responsible for causing such pain. From this information, we have only just begun to learn the keys to prevention.

However, strengthening the torso has always been an important part of Qigong practice in China. From past experience, it is understood that if the physical torso is not strong and the Qi circulation is not abundant in the center, the immune system will be weak and a person can sicken easily. On one hand, Qigong teaches a practitioner how to build up the Qi and, with the coordination of the breathing, use the mind to enhance its circulation; on the other hand, it emphasizes the health of the physical body.

In the next section, we will discuss in more detail how Qigong massage and exercise can prevent and cure back pain. We will also summarize the differences between Chinese Qigong massage and exercise from the techniques of the West.

5-3. How Can Qigong Cure Back Pain?

Due to a lack of knowledge and experience in acupuncture and herbal treatments in general, I will not include these two fields in our discussion. If you are interested in knowing more about the treatments from these two fields, you should refer to other related books and documents. In this section, the discussion will be limited to Qigong massage and exercise.

In Chinese medicine, the concept of Qi is used both in the diagnosis and in treatment. A basic principle of Chinese medicine is that **you have to re-balance the Qi before you can cure the root of a disease. Only then can you also repair the physical damage and rebuild your physical strength and health**. This theory is very simple. Your entire body is made up of living cells. When these cells receive the proper Qi supply, they will function normally and even repair themselves. However, if the Qi supply is abnormal and this condition persists, then even though the cells were originally healthy, they will become damaged or changed (perhaps even becoming cancerous). In light of this basic Qi theory, let us first discuss why Qigong can be effective in curing back pain. Then we will explain how Chinese Qigong exercises and massage reach this goal.

Why Qigong is Effective for Back Pain

Qigong Maintains and Increases Smooth Qi Circulation. As mentioned earlier, the goal of Qigong healing is to re-establish a strong, smooth flow of Qi through the affected area. When this happens, physical damage can be repaired and strength rebuilt. Chinese physicians have always believed that as long as you are alive, physical damage to the body can be repaired through improving the Qi and blood circulation. Most Western physicians don't agree with this, and damage to some deep parts of the body—for example, the osteoarthritis caused by aging and the degeneration of the joints—cannot be reversed. However, some Western physicians are beginning to change their minds about this.[2]

Qigong Strengthens the Physical and Mental Bodies. The greatest benefit of Chinese Qigong is probably in the physical (Yang) and mental (Yin) training. Qigong teaches you how to regulate your mind to a calm, profound and concentrated meditative state. It also teaches you how to use your regulated mind in coordination with deep breathing to lead the Qi circulating in your body. From this internal guidance and coordination with specific Qigong movements, you can either heal yourself or rebuild the strength of your physical body. From the Yin (mental body) and Yang (physical body) balance, you regain your health.

Qigong Strengthens the Immune and Hormone Production Systems. Western science knows that the body's immune system is closely related to the endocrine glands, which produce hormones. Hormones, as they are now understood, do not actually create processes. What they do, however, is cause the fundamental processes such as growth, reproduction and sex to speed up or slow down. (The word *hormone* comes from a Greek word which means to excite, to stimulate or to stir up.) They also strengthen the ability of the immune system to fight diseases. For example, it is believed that the thymus gland (which is located just behind the top of the sternum) plays an important role in the body's immune system. Exactly how this happens is still not completely understood. We still do not know very much about the pineal gland in the upper back part of the brain, nor do we have a full understanding of the function of the thymus.[3] In fact, it has only recently come to be believed that hormone production is significantly related to the aging process.

Many of us know of people who were deathly sick, but who had a very high spirit and a strong desire to survive, and miraculously recovered. Both Western and Eastern religions tell of many such cases. Chinese Qigong practitioners believe that if a sick person can lead Qi to the brain through concentration or through strong desire, he or she can evoke a powerful healing force. A possible explanation is that the stronger Qi flow activates the pineal and pituitary glands so that they generate more hormones. We now know that the most important function of the pituitary gland is to stimulate, regulate and coordinate the functions of the other endocrine glands.[3] For this reason it is sometimes called the "master gland."

In Chinese Qigong, the Upper Dan Tian (which some Westerners refer to as the "third eye") is considered the center of your whole being. If you raise your spirit, which resides there, you can energize your body, manifest amazing physical and mental strength, and recover more quickly from injury or sickness. Certain groups in the West have also recognized its importance as the center of the spirit, and consider it a "third eye," which is able to sense further than the physical eyes can see.

If we combine the understanding of old and new, East and West, we can conclude that what actually happens, probably because of mental concentration, is that a stronger current of bioelectricity is led to the pineal and pituitary glands to activate the production of hormones. This stimulates the entire endocrine system and causes it to function more effectively, improving healing, cellular regeneration, reproduction and growth. If this is correct, then it is possible to begin a new era of scientific self-healing or spiritual healing. An alternative result is that we may learn how to devise electrical equipment to activate the pineal and pituitary glands to improve the effectiveness and speed of healing. Perhaps we may also be able to find the secret key to slowing down the aging process.

Qigong Raises the Spirit of Vitality. The spirit is closely tied to the mind, and cannot be separated from it. In Qigong practice, the mind is considered the general in the battle against sickness. When the mind (general) has a strong will, thoroughly understands the battlefield (the body), wisely and carefully sets up the strategy (the breathing technique), and effectively and efficiently manages the soldiers (the Qi), then the morale (spirit) of the general and soldiers can be high. When this happens, sickness can be conquered and health regained.

When you use Qigong to treat your back pain, you must first treat your mind by changing the way you look at your sickness and your life. The first thing you need to do is to stop passively accepting the negative things that have happened to you. Become more active and take charge of your life. Most basically, learn how to keep the back pain from disturbing your peace of mind. Remember, doing something is better than doing nothing. Second, you must rebuild your confidence in your ability to treat your back pain. Even though you may have failed before, don't let that discourage you. Learn about the causes of your problem, understand the theory of this new treatment, and try to think about how you can make the treatment more effective. Once you do this, you will have rebuilt your confidence not only in the treatment, but also in your life.

Once you have built up your confidence, the third thing you need to do is to develop the willpower, patience and perseverance needed to keep up the treatment. The best way to prevent back pain from returning once you have cured it is to make Qigong part of your life. Fourth, after you have practiced Qigong for a while, you will understand your body better and you will deal with such problems more easily. You may realize that the pain is not necessarily all bad. Pain draws your attention to your body and helps you to understand yourself better. Pain can also help you to build up willpower and perseverance. However, you must first know what pain is, only then will you stop it. This is called "regulating your mind." Remember that medicine is only a temporary solution.

You can see that Chinese Qigong heals by going to the root of the problem. It improves the entire body, both mentally and physically, and strengthens the immune system. Only when this is done will the illness be healed completely.

How Chinese Qigong Exercises Differ from Western Exercises

1. From a theoretical point of view, Qigong originated from the concept of regulating the Qi (from an imbalanced condition into a balanced one) both before and after any physical damage has occurred. Western medicine, however,

does not yet fully accept the existence of Qi or bioelectricity, and is therefore not concerned with it.

2. Chinese Qigong considers the regulation of the body to be the most basic and important factor in successful practice. Regulating the body means to bring your body into a very relaxed, centered and balanced state. Only then can your mind be calm and comfortable. When the body is relaxed, the Qi can circulate freely and be led easily anywhere you wish, such as to the skin or even deep into the bone marrow and the internal organs. To cure back pain, you have to be so relaxed that you can lead the Qi deep into the joint where it can repair the damage. Western back pain exercises are not usually specifically concerned with relaxation.

    The first priority in Qigong exercise for back pain is learning how to relax and avoid muscle/tendon tension and stress in the joint area, which is especially critical in severe cases of back pain. Chinese physicians reason that exercises which tense the muscles and tendons will inhibit the Qi circulation from going deep into the damaged joint. Furthermore, **tension of the muscles and tendons increases pressure on the joint and can increase the damage**. Therefore, Chinese physicians recommend relaxed, gentle movements first to smoothly increase the Qi circulation. Only when the patient has rebuilt the strength of the joint will the muscles and tendons be exercised. After all, strong muscles and tendons are what will prevent future joint damage.

    However, in Western physical exercise for back pain, before any healing or rehabilitation of the deep joint area is done, strenuous muscle and tendon strengthening exercises have already been conducted. To a Chinese Qigong practitioner, knowing the correct way of exercising from soft to hard is a key to rebuilding the healthy condition of the joints from deep within to the surface.

3. With Qigong, in addition to the body being relaxed, the breathing must be long, deep and calm. According to Qigong theory, breathing is the strategy of your practice. When you exhale, you instinctively and naturally lead Qi to the surface of your body, and when you inhale, you lead it inward to the bone marrow and the internal organs. In Qigong you have to learn to breathe deeply and calmly in coordination with your thinking. This way, your mind can lead the Qi strongly into the damaged area. In Western back pain exercise, coordinating the deep breathing with the movement is not emphasized.

4. In the first chapter, we explained that since the mind is one of the major forces (EMF) of Qi or bioelectric circulation, it has an important role in healing. In order to make your Qigong practice really effective, in addition to regulating your body and breathing, you must also regulate your mind. Regulating your mind means to lead it away from outside distractions and turn it toward feeling what is going on inside your body. In order to lead Qi

to the damaged places in your body, your mind must be calm, relaxed, and concentrated, so that you can feel or sense the Qi. The mind, therefore, plays a very important role in Qigong. Western back pain exercise, on the other hand, is usually not concerned at all with the training of the meditative mind.

5. Another significant difference between Qigong and Western back pain exercise is that Qigong emphasizes not only healing the joints, but also rebuilding the health of the internal organs. Remember, only when the internal organs are healthy can the root of the Qi imbalance be removed and, therefore, the cause of the sickness be corrected. But Qigong is not just concerned with bringing the organs back to health, it also works to strengthen them. Western back pain exercises, in contrast, are not at all concerned with the health of the internal organs.

6. One of the most significant results of Qigong practice is maintaining hormone production at a healthy level, which keeps the immune system functioning effectively. In Western medicine, imbalanced hormone production is adjusted with drugs.

7. The most significant difference between Qigong and Western back pain exercise is probably that practicing Qigong draws the patient gradually into an acquaintance with the inner energy side of his or her body. In other words, internal self-awareness will be increased. Once this is experienced, patients can start to feel energy imbalances when they are just beginning, and consequently can correct them before physical damage occurs. In fact, this is the key to preventing most illnesses.

You can see that, although many of the movements of Qigong and Western back pain exercises are similar, the theory of Qigong is more profound and therefore the challenge is more significant. In fact, the best way to maintain your health and rebuild your Qi and body is by understanding the theory of Qigong and starting the training. If you are interested in knowing more about Qigong training, please refer to the book: *The Root of Chinese Qigong*, from YMAA Publication Center.

Because this book will also introduce Qigong massage for back pain, we would like to point out some of the major differences between Qigong massage and regular Western massage.

How Chinese Qigong Massage Differs from Western Massage

1. Chinese massage pays attention to improving the circulation of both Qi and blood, while Western massage normally emphasizes only good blood circulation and a comfortable, easy feeling.

2. In Chinese massage, the masseur (or masseuse) and the patient must communicate with each other both through touch and through deeper levels of contact. This mutual cooperation enables the masseur to use his or her mind

to either lead Qi into the patient or to remove excess Qi from the patient's body. Therefore, Qigong massage requires a higher level of experience and training in concentration. This means that the massage is not limited to only a physical massage, it is also a Qi massage. The most important part of this cooperation is that the patient can use his or her own mind to relax the area being massaged and make the massage more effective. Furthermore, this cooperation helps the patient to calm the mind and relax deeply into the internal organs and bone marrow, which makes it possible for the massage to regulate the Qi. In Western massage, coordination between the masseur and the patient is not emphasized.

3. Cavity press or acupressure techniques are considered part of Qigong massage. Like Japanese Shiatsu massage, which is derived from Chinese acupressure, finger pressure on the cavities is used to regulate the Qi circulation and to remove Qi and blood stagnation in the affected areas. To do this kind of massage effectively requires not only that the masseur know the location of the cavities, but that he or she also understand the twelve Qi channels, how to use them to remove excess Qi from affected areas and how to bring in nourishing Qi. It is also extremely helpful if the masseur is experienced in Qigong. This kind of practice is almost completely ignored in Western massage.

References

1. *The Body Electric*, by Dr. Robert O. Becker, MD., and Gary Selden, 1985. William Morrow and Company, Inc., 105 Madison Ave., New York, 10016.

2. "Keeping the Human Body Active Reduces Risk of Osteoarthritis," by Dr. Gifford-Jones, *Toronto Globe and Mail,* January 31, 1989.

3. *The Complete Medical Guide*, Benjamin F. Miller, M.D., Simon and Schuster, New York, 1978.

CHAPTER 6

Qigong for Back Pain

氣功防治腰酸背疼

6-1. Introduction

Before proceeding any further, we would first like to discuss the attitude you must have in your practice. Quite frequently, people who are ill are reluctant to get involved in the healing process. This is especially true for back pain patients. Both Western and Chinese physicians have had difficulty persuading them to get involved in regular exercise or Qigong. The main reason for this reluctance is that the patients are afraid of pain, and therefore believe that these kinds of exercise are harmful. In order to conquer this obstacle to your healing, you must understand the theory of healing and the reason for practicing. Only then will you have the confidence necessary for continued practice. Remember, **a physician may have an excellent prescription for your illness, but if you don't take the medicine, it won't do you any good.**

Another factor that has caused the failure of many a potential cure is laziness. Because the healing process is very slow, it is very easy to become **impatient and lazy**. Very often in life we will know exactly what it is that we need to do, but because we are controlled by the emotional parts of our minds, we end up either not doing what we need to, or not doing it right. Either way, our efforts have all been in vain.

It seems that most of the time our "emotional mind" (Xin, 心) and "wisdom mind" (Yi, 意) are in opposition. In China there is a proverb that says: "You are your own biggest enemy." This means that your emotional mind often wants to go in the opposite direction from what your wisdom mind knows is best. If your wisdom mind is able to conquer and govern your emotional mind, then there is nothing that can stop you from doing anything you want. Usually, however, your emotional mind makes you lazy, causes you to feel embarrassment (i.e., put a mask on your face), and destroys your willpower and perseverance. We always know that our clear-headed wisdom mind understands what needs to be done, but too often we surrender to our emotional mind and becomes a slave of our emotions. When this happens, we usually feel guilty deep down in our hearts, and we try to find a good excuse so that we won't have to feel so guilty.

The first step when you decide to practice Qigong is to strengthen your wisdom mind and use it to govern your emotional mind. Only then will you have enough patience and perseverance to keep practicing. You can see that the **first key to successful training is not the techniques themselves but rather your self-control**. I sincerely believe that as long as you have strong will, patience, and perseverance, there is nothing that can't be accomplished.

Forming the habit of practicing regularly actually represents changing your life style. Once you have started regulating your life through Qigong, it can not only cure your back pain and re-strengthen your spine, but it can also keep you healthy and make both your mental and physical lives much happier.

In this chapter, we will introduce some Qigong practices which have been experienced and proven to have great success in curing and/or preventing back pain. Although there are four fields of Chinese treatment for back pain, as mentioned earlier, since I am not qualified nor experienced in the area of herbal and acupuncture treatments, I will only focus on Qigong exercise and massage. Still, I would like to remind you that among the four Chinese treatment methods, though the other methods can alleviate pain, only Qigong exercise is able to re-strengthen and rebuild the **strong root** of the healthy spine.

In the next section, we will first review the important training procedures and keys which we have discussed in the first chapter. Without understanding these essential keys to training, the effectiveness of your practice will be shallow. In section 6-3, Qigong exercises for back pain will be introduced for the reconditioning of your back. If you have a hard time learning these movements, you may also obtain a videotape which will demonstrate the movements clearly. Finally, in the last section of this chapter, massage techniques and cavities will be introduced.

6-2. Important Training Keys

In this section, we will first review the five important regulating procedures for successful Qigong training which we discussed in the first chapter. Understanding these five factors profoundly will lead you to an in-depth level of practice. Naturally, the results will also be much greater.

After this, we will summarize some important keys for Qigong practice. In you can comprehend these keys, you will have grasped the secret of Qigong practice.

Five Regulatings (Wu Tiao, 五調)

Regulating the Body. Before you start your Qigong exercises, you should first calm down your mind and use this mind to bring your body into a calm and relaxed state. Naturally, you should always be concerned with your mental and physical centers. Only then will you be able to find your balance. When you have both mental and physical relaxation, centering and balance, you will be both natural and comfortable. This is the key to regulating your body.

When you relax, you should learn to relax deeply into your internal organs, and especially the muscles which enclose the organs. In addition, you must also place your mind on the joints that are giving you trouble. The more you can bring your mind deep into the joint and relax it, the more Qi will circulate smoothly and freely to repair the damage.

Regulating the Breathing. As mentioned before, breathing is the central strategy in Qigong practice. According to Qigong theory, when you inhale you lead Qi inward and when you exhale you lead Qi outward. This is our natural instinct. For example, when you feel cold in the wintertime, in order to keep from loosing Qi out of your body you naturally inhale more than you exhale to lead the Qi inward, which also closes the pores in the skin. However, in the summertime when you are too hot you naturally exhale more than you inhale in order to lead Qi out of your body. When you do this you start to sweat and the pores open.

In Qigong practice, generally, you want to lead the Qi to the internal organs and bone marrow, so you must learn how to use inhalation to lead the Qi inward. In addition, you would also like to lead the Qi outward to the skin surface and beyond to strengthen your Guardian Qi and therefore protect yourself from the negative Qi influences around you.

When you use Qigong to cure your back pain, you must learn how to inhale and exhale deeply and calmly so that you can lead the Qi deep into the joints, and also outward to dissipate the excess or stagnant Qi which has accumulated in the joints. Therefore, in addition to relaxing when you practice, you should always remember to inhale and exhale deeply. When you inhale, place your mind deep in the joint, and when you exhale, lead the Qi to the surface of the skin.

There are more than ten different methods of breathing in Chinese Qigong practice. However, there are only two which are commonly used in our daily life. One is called "Normal Abdominal Breathing" or "Buddhist Breathing," and the other is called "Reversed Abdominal Breathing" or "Daoist Breathing."

In **Normal Abdominal Breathing, when you inhale, the abdomen is gently pushed out and when you exhale, the abdomen is withdrawn** (Figures 6-1 and 6-2). In order to fill up the Qi to an abundant level in the lower abdominal area, **when you inhale you should also gently push your Huiyin (Co-1, 會陰) cavity (or anus) out and when you exhale, you hold it up gently** (Figure 6-3). Remember, you **should not** tense this area during either inhalation or exhalation unless you are doing some special training such as Hard Qigong. Tension in this area can only make the Qi circulation stagnant in Small Circulation practice.

In **Reverse Abdominal Breathing, when you inhale, the abdomen is gently pulled inward, and when you exhale the abdomen is gently pushed outward** (Figures 6-4 and 6-5). Again, the coordination of the Huiyin (Co-1) cavity (or anus) is very important. The Huiyin (i.e., Meeting Yin) cavity is a major gate which regulates the four Yin vessels, and therefore controls the Qi status of the body. Traditionally,

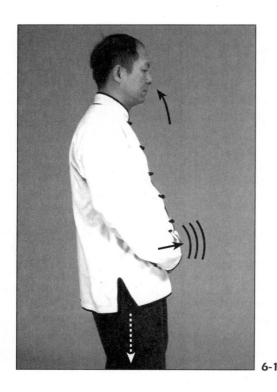 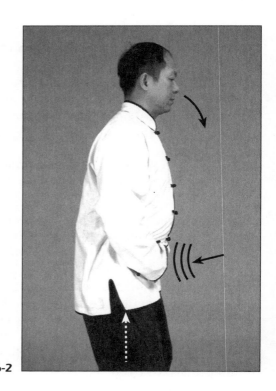

6-1   6-2

a master would not reveal this secret of Huiyin control to any student until he was completely trusted by the master.

When you practice **Reverse Abdominal Breathing, as you inhale you should gently pull your Huiyin (Co-1) cavity (or anus) up, and as you exhale you should gently push it out**. Again, you **should not** tense this area during either inhalation or exhalation unless you are doing some special training such as Hard Qigong.

Often, a Qigong beginner will mistakenly believe that Reverse Abdominal Breathing is not natural. On the contrary, Reverse Abdominal Breathing is one of our normal breathing habits. Normally, if your emotions are not disturbed or you do not have any intention to energize your muscular power to a higher manifestation of power, you use Normal Breathing. However, when your emotional mind is disturbed, you may change your breathing into Reverse Breathing without realizing it. For example, when you are happy and laugh, you exhale while making the sound of "*Ha*," and your abdominal area pushes out. When you are sad and cry, you inhale while making the sound of "*Hen*," and your abdomen is withdrawn. Also, when you are scared, you inhale while holding your abdomen inward.

As mentioned previously, another occasion in which you use Reverse Breathing is when you have an intention to energize your muscular power to a higher, more powerful and spiritual state. For example, if you are pushing a car or lifting a heavy weight, you will use Reverse Breathing. In order to manifest your power to a higher level in martial arts, you must train your Reverse Breathing technique to be more efficient. This is the secret of Jin and the way of Dao.

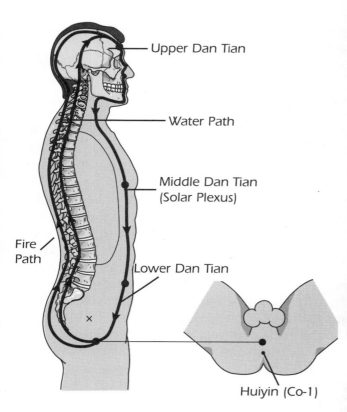

Upper Dan Tian

Water Path

Middle Dan Tian
(Solar Plexus)

Fire
Path

Lower Dan Tian

Huiyin (Co-1)

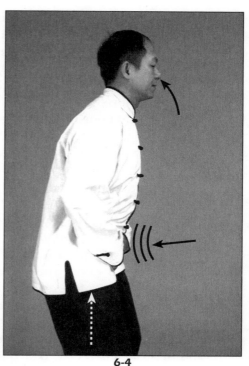

6-4

Figure 6-3. The Huiyin Cavity (Co-1)

Often, a Qigong or martial arts beginner encounters the problem of tightness in the abdominal area. The reason for this is that in Reverse Breathing, when you inhale the diaphragm is pulling downward while the abdominal area is withdrawing. This can generate tension in the stomach area. To reduce this problem, you must start on a small scale with Reverse Breathing, and only after you can control the muscles in the abdominal area efficiently, gradually relax the area and eliminate the problem. Naturally, this will take time.

Regulating the Mind. In Qigong, the mind is considered the general who directs the battle against sickness. After all, it is your mind which manages all of your thinking and activity.

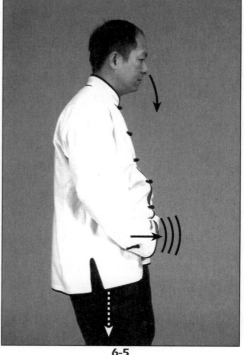

6-5

Therefore, a clear calm mind is very important so that you can judge clearly and accurately. In addition, your mind must also be concentrated. Your mind can generate an EMF (an electromotive force or "voltage difference") which causes your Qi to circulate. The more you concentrate, the stronger you can lead the Qi.

When you have a calm and concentrated mind, you can feel and sense the problem correctly. Therefore, when you practice Qigong for your back pain you must learn how to bring your mind inward so that you can understand the situation, and you must use your concentrated mind to lead the Qi.

In practice, when you regulate your mind, you must, at the same time, coordinate with your breathing. If your breathing is deep and calm, your mind can be led to a profound meditative state. Moreover, normally when you inhale longer than you exhale, you can calm down easily. The other side of the token is that if you exhale longer than you inhale, you will be excited and lead the mind outside of your body.

Therefore, in order to lead your mind into your body, you must calm down and inhale deeply and slenderly, while physically becoming extremely relaxed. Once you can calm down your mind, you should then bring it to your third eye (or Upper Dan Tian), located on your forehead. From both Chinese and Western ancient spiritual cultivation experience, it is recognized that paying attention to this spot is a way to lead your mind from outside of your body to an inner awareness. The reason for this is that it is believed that our conscious mind (i.e., spirit) resides here.

If you practice correctly, you will soon feel that as you breathe, this place is harmonizing with your breathing. You will feel warmth and a very little pressure on this spot. If you can pay attention to this place for a few minutes, you will gradually lead your mind to an awareness of your inner feelings.

Next, you move your mind from your third eye to your sternum. As mentioned earlier, this area is considered to be the Middle Dan Tian, which accumulates the fire Qi. In Chinese Qigong, it is believed that the fire Qi at the Middle Dan Tian will make you excited and emotional. Therefore, in order to lead your mind to a deeper and calmer meditative state, you must learn how to calm down the fire at the Middle Dan Tian. Therefore, you inhale deeply and use your mind to lead the Qi from the Middle Dan Tian to the lungs and when you exhale, simply relax your lungs. The lungs are considered to be Metal in Chinese five element medical philosophy. Metal is able to lead the heat away and therefore cool down the fire. That is why whenever we are excited, if we inhale deeply and then relax, we can calm down easily. Through this breathing practice, you will have cooled off your excited energy, which is the key trick to leading your mind to the second phase of deep meditation.

Finally, lead your mind to your Lower Dan Tian and keep there for a while with the coordination of deep breathing. This will help you clam down to the deepest possible meditative state. When you are in this state, your mind will be very clear and feel what is happening in your body. If you are interested in knowing more about how to use your mind to lead both your mental and physical bodies into a deeply relaxed and meditative state, you may refer to the book: *The Essence of Shaolin White Crane*, and the audio tape: *Self Relaxation*, from YMAA Publication Center.

Regulating the Qi. Once you have regulated your body, breathing, and mind, you will already be in a good condition to start regulating your Qi, and can lead your Qi anywhere in your body to make repairs.

If you have an injury or some damage which you need to repair, you should first inhale and use your mind to lead the Qi deeply into that area, then exhale and again use your mind to lead the Qi away from the place. If you do this correctly, you will soon feel this place grow warm with a sensational feeling which coordinates with your breathing.

Regulating the Spirit. The final key to Qigong is raising your spirit of vitality. Good morale or fighting spirit is necessary to win the fight against illness. When your spirit is high, your willpower is strong, your mind is firm, and your patience can last long. In addition, when your spirit is high your emotions are under control and your wisdom mind can be calm and lead the Qi to circulate in the body more efficiently. This will significantly reduce the time for healing.

You should now have a clear idea of how to practice most efficiently. During the course of your practice you should frequently remind yourself of these key requirements. If you would like to learn more about these keys to Qigong practice, you may refer to the book: *The Root of Chinese Qigong*, from YMAA Publication Center.

Important Keys to Practice

Here we will list a few important keys to practice. These keys originated from many ancient Qigong masters after their life-time of experience. Naturally, most of these keys are closely related or linked with the five regulatings discussed above.

Balance of Body and Heart (Emotional Mind) (Shen Xin Ping Heng, 身心平衡). In Chinese Qigong, a human has two bodies, the physical body and the Qi (energy) body. When these two bodies are harmonized and united with each other, you will be healthy and the spirit can be raised. In order to reach this goal, you must first regulate your mind. That means you should learn how to use your wisdom mind (Yi, 意) to govern your emotional mind (Xin, 心). Only then can your mind be calm and remain emotionally neutral. Under these conditions, your judgment can be accurate. When you use this clear mind to balance your physical and Qi body's conditions, they can work together and coordinate with each other harmoniously.

Unification of Internal and External (Nei Wai He Yi, 內外合一). When you use a clear and wise mind to make a good judgment, both your physical body (external), mind (internal), and Qi (internal) will all work together as one unit. However, even this does not mean that they can harmonize with each other. Only when they are harmonized can mutual coordination be achieved and the spirit of life be heightened. When you reach this stage, it is called "Nei Wai Xie He" (內外諧合), which means "mutual harmonization of internal and external."

In order to reach this level, you must first learn how to regulate your mind and bring it into the internal feeling of your body. If your mind cannot be restrained internally, you will not be able to feel any physical problem or Qi imbalance in your body. This kind of practice is called: "Nei Shi Fan Ting" (內視返聽), which means "to see internally and to listen inwardly." Since it will take a great deal of patience and time to train this, it is also called: "Nei Shi Gongfu" (內視功夫), which means "Gongfu of internal vision."

If we apply the above concepts to our Qigong healing for back pain, we must first educate our mind to understand the structure of our physical body, especially in the lower back area. From this understanding, we can comprehend the problem and know the situation clearly. Moreover, our mind must also be able to feel the Qi imbalance in our body. Once your mind knows both the physical body (Yang) and the Qi body (Yin) clearly, then you can adopt the treatments wisely to solve any problem.

To make the healing most effective, you should not only just learn the techniques. More important is that, through your mind's coordination, you make your physical body and Qi body harmonize with each other smoothly. When this happens, the healing process will be fast and effective.

In order to harmonize the external with the internal, you must first learn how to regulate your body and perform the movements smoothly. When it is necessary to be relaxed, you are relaxed and when it is necessary to be tensed, you are tensed adequately. If you can do this, then you can adjust the depth of healing according to your inner feeling and understanding.

In addition, you must also learn how to use your mind to govern your breathing and coordinate with your external physical movements. Once you have reached a high level of coordination and harmonization of your mind, physical body, breathing, and Qi body, you will have accomplished 90 percent of healing.

Mutual Dependence of Heart (Mind) and Breathing (Xin Xi Xiang Yi, 心息相依). In order to reach the final harmonization of the physical body and the Qi body, your mind must always pay attention to your breathing. Breathing is considered to be the strategy. When the strategy is correct, the action can be effective and the result can be fruitful. If your mind and breathing are coordinating with each other smoothly, the Qi can be lead effectively, naturally, and smoothly.

Use the Yi (Wisdom Mind) to Lead the Qi (Yi Yi Yin Qi, 以意引氣). Once you have a good coordination of your physical body and Qi body, then you learn how to use your mind to lead the Qi. Naturally, the first step is learning how to keep your mind at the Lower Dan Tian (bioelectric battery) located at your physical center. When your mind is able to stay in this center anytime you want, then physically you have a balance on the top and bottom, left and right, and front and rear. Not only that, the distribution of Qi will also be balanced. When you are in this centered state, you are relaxed and mentally neutral. This practice is called: "Yi Shou Dan Tian" (意守丹田), which means "(wisdom) mind is kept at Dan Tian." This is the process of learning how to preserve the Qi and store it in the human battery without wasting it. Theoretically speaking, the more you learn how to conserve your Qi, the longer your vital force can last.

The next step is learning how to use the mind to lead the Qi to repair physical damage. It is believed in Chinese medicine that as long as we provide the right condition for the cells to multiply, any physical damage in our body can be repaired. The first requirement is to provide plenty of Qi. Without this Qi, the repair will be slow or non-existent.

The trick to using the mind to lead the Qi is in the spirit (Shen). It is known in Chinese Qigong society that when the spirit is high, the Qi can be led efficiently. Spirit is like the morale of a soldier. When morale is high, the soldier's fighting capability and potential is high. That is why it is said: "Yi Shen Yu Qi" (以神馭氣), which means "use the Shen to govern the Qi." It is also said: "Yi is on the spirit of vitality, not on Qi, (if) or Qi, (circulation of Qi) will be stagnant."[1]

The way of building up your spirit is to first establish your positive attitude; that means your confidence and strong will. Without these two factors, you will not be able to conquer sickness.

6-3. Qigong Exercises for Back Pain

Out of all the Chinese martial Qigong developed in the last fifteen hundred years, there are only a few styles which pay attention to the torso's strength, especially the spine. These styles are: White Crane, Snake, Dragon, and Taijiquan. The reason for this is simply that these styles are classified as either soft or soft-hard styles of martial arts in China. In order to manifest martial power softly and strongly, the condition of the spine is critical. Without the strong foundation of the torso, not only will power not be manifested forcefully, but spinal injury may also be experienced.

It is because of the above reason that, since ancient times, these styles have been recognized as having the best Qigong exercises for spinal conditioning. Many Chinese physicians have since adopted these Qigong practices as a way of spinal rehabilitation for those patients with spine problems.

At this point, you may be curious as to why so many Qigong healing exercises were developed in Chinese martial arts society, especially in the Buddhist and Daoist martial arts monasteries. If we examine Chinese martial arts history, we can see that often Chinese martial artists were training in the deep mountains with masters. Since there was usually no doctor in the deep mountains, whenever there was an injury, the martial artists needed to take care of it by themselves. After few thousand years of self healing practice, Chinese martial artists became experts in treating injury and have been recognized as one of the highest authorities on many kinds of injury treatments in Chinese medical society. The common treatments are massage, herbs, and/or Qigong exercises.

The Qigong exercises introduced in this section are mainly from White Crane and Taijiquan martial arts. The reason for this is simply that these are the two styles with which I am most familiar. It is well known that the key to becoming an expert is to practice continuously, to ponder and to accumulate experience. Experience is the best teacher. As long as you remain humble, ponder and combine theory and practice, you will soon become an expert in dealing with spinal problems. If you are interested in knowing more about White Crane and Taiji Qigong, please refer to the books: *The Essence of Shaolin White Crane* and *The Essence of Tai Chi Chi Kung*, from YMAA Publication Center.

Qigong Exercises

External Qigong is also called "Wai Dan" (external elixir, 外丹) Qigong, since it emphasizes external physical movements and/or uses the mind to lead the Qi to the extremities or local areas of the body either for healing or physical strengthening. External Qigong can be classified as soft, soft-hard and hard. In the soft category, the muscles and tendons are relaxed to a deep level while the joints are moved. The main purpose of this soft external Qigong is that, through repeating the movements, **the ligaments are exercised and the blood circulation deep in the joints is improved**.

Soft-hard external Qigong moves the joints softly, while twisting the joints or slightly tensing the tendons in the joint areas. The main purpose of this Qigong is **to strengthen the structure of the joints, such as ligaments and tendons**. Again, through repeating the movements, the joints are conditioned gradually. Any injury in the joints can be repaired due to the enhanced Qi and blood circulation.

Finally, hard external Qigong is used to **build up the strength and endurance of the muscles and tendons**. Normally, only the physical tension can be seen externally. This Qigong is not too different from weight lifting. The only difference is the use of the mind. In Qigong, the mind is used to lead the Qi to the muscular body first before it is tensed. From this mind and body coordination, the efficiency and effectiveness of the exercises can be enhanced to a higher level. As mentioned earlier, this is called the "unification of the internal and external."

According to past experience, in order to improve the Qi and blood circulation in the deep places of the joints, we must **first loosen up the joints**. After loosening up the joints, a **gentle and firm stretching** should follow in order to open up the joints, especially if there is any injury or pain in them. Then, **correct joint movements** should be done repeatedly until the joints are warm. Finally, **joint loosening exercises** should be used to lead the Qi away from the joints.

Next, we will introduce Qigong exercises for back pain. Before you start, you should recognize an important fact. After your exercise, you may discover and experience that your back or torso muscles are more sore and painful than before. This is quite normal. There are two reasons for this. First, you are exercising muscles and tendons which you seldom exercised before. Their condition is weak. Therefore, you should start the following exercises with only a few repetitions at first. Only if you feel stronger should you increase the number of repetitions. That means you are **conditioning your physical body from weak to strong**.

Second, after you exercise, the circulation of the Qi and blood will be enhanced. This will enliven your nervous system at the local area and make it more sensitive. When this happens, you will experience soreness. You should not be discouraged by this. Treat it as a challenge. Remember, the more you move, the better your physical condition will become. However, should you feel sharp pain, burning and/or tingling or a pain which radiates down into your legs, you should again reduce the number of repetitions and consult with your doctor.

Loosening up the Lower Back

1. Place both arms in front of your chest with palms facing downward. Then, turn your body from side to side gently (Figure 6-6). This will loosen up the torso muscles and gradually excite them. Repeat about six times each side.

2. Continue to keep both your arms right in front of your chest. Loosening up your torso by moving your hips forward to generate an upward wave motion while circling both your arms up, forward and then downward continuously (Figure 6-7). The intention of this movement is to move the torso gently to loosen up the muscles.

3. Place your hands on your waist and then circle your waist horizontally (Figure 6-8). First, circle to one side a few times and then to the other side. If you have already experienced pain, make the circle smaller. However, if you feel comfortable without too much pain, you may increase the size of the circular motion and also the number of circles. This will loosen up the lower back area and the hip joints. Only you can decide how big the circle should be. The main goal is to loosen up any tightness in the waist area caused from back pain. When you are doing the above loosening up exercises, you should breath naturally. **Do not hold your breath**. Holding you breath will make your muscles tense.

Stretching

After you have loosened up your waist area, you should stretch your torso. If you stretch your torso correctly, you can stimulate the cells into an excited state, and this will improve Qi and blood circulation. This is the key to maintaining the health of the physical body. However, when you stretch you should treat your muscles, tendons and ligaments like a rubber band. Stretch gently and gradually. If you stretch too much and too fast, you will break the rubber band. For muscles, tendons and ligaments, that means the tearing off of fibers. However, if you under stretch, it will not be effective. A good stretch should feel comfortable and stimulating.

1. Stretching the Torso (Shuang Shou Tuo Tian, 雙手托天). First, interlock your fingers and lift your hands up over your head while imagining that you are pushing upward with your hands and pushing downward with your feet (Figure 6-9). Do not tense your muscles; because this will constrict your body and prevent you from stretching. If you do this stretch correctly, you will feel the muscles in your waist area tensing slightly because they are being pulled simultaneously from the top and the bottom. Next, use your mind to relax and stretch out a little bit more. Remember to keep your palms turned directly upward, don't allow them to roll toward the front. Also, be careful not to thrust out the lower ribs, and keep your pelvis level. After you have stretched

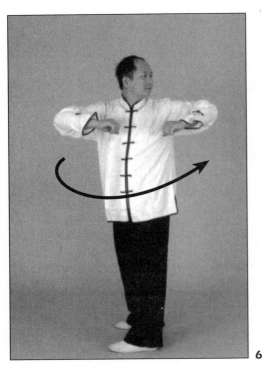
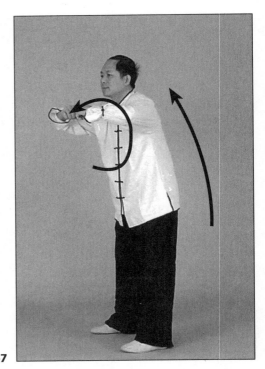

6-6   6-7

for about ten seconds, twist your upper body to one side to twist the trunk muscles (Figure 6-10). Stay to the side for three to five seconds, turn your body to face forward and then turn to the other side. Stay there for three to five seconds. Repeat the upper body twisting three times, come back to the center, and tilt your upper body to the side and stay there for about three to five seconds (Figure 6-11), then tilt to the other side. Again repeat three times, maintaining the feeling of stretching upward throughout the entire process. Next, bend forward gently and use your pelvis to wave the hips from side to side to loosen up the lower spine (Figure 6-12). Stay there for ten seconds. Finally, if possible, squat down with your feet flat on the ground to stretch your ankles (Figure 6-13) and then lift your heels up to stretch the toes (Figure 6-14). Repeat the entire process three times. After you finish, the inside of your body should feel very comfortable and warm.

When you practice the above stretching, you should not hold your breath. Once you hold your breath, your body will be more tense. How far you should stretch depends on your feeling. If you feel only slight pain and discomfort, it is good. However, if you feel the pain is too much, producing both physical tension and mental disturbance, then you may have pushed too far. Proceed cautiously and gently, and push a little bit farther each time. You are looking for progress, but without feeling uncomfortable pain.

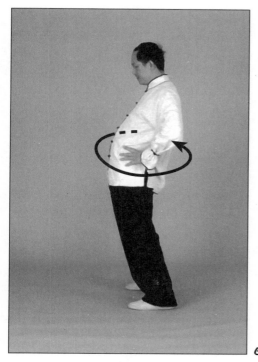
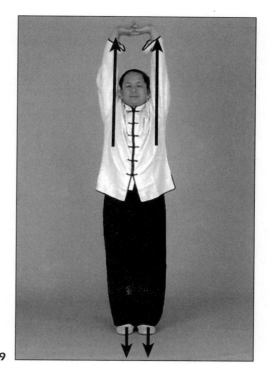

6-8   6-9

If you are in good health already and are looking for a more aggressive stretch to reach the ligaments, then when your arms are up above your head, keep the torso stretched while circling your waist area (Figure 6-15). Try six circulations to each side at the beginning. Remember, too much exercise may cause injury and too little will not be effective. You are the one who should make the judgment.

2. **Stretching and Loosening up the Neck (Bai He Shen Jing, Na Zha Tan Hai, 白鶴伸頸，哪吒探海).** After you have stretched your torso, next you should stretch your neck. The neck is the junction of the blood and Qi exchanging path between the head and the body. Whenever the neck is stiffened or the spine in the neck is injured, this blood and Qi exchange will be stagnant. Consequently, your brain will not have proper nourishment. In addition, the muscles in the neck extend downward to the chest and the back. Whenever the back is tense, the neck is also stiff and vice versa. Therefore, in order to maintain your health and relieve back tension, you must also learn the correct manner of loosening up your neck, including the muscles, tendons and ligaments.

First, you should stretch the muscles and tendons around the neck and gradually reach to the ligaments, which are hidden deeply between the joints. To stretch the neck muscles and tendons, you should focus on the four biggest

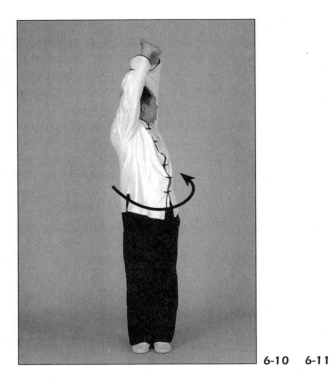

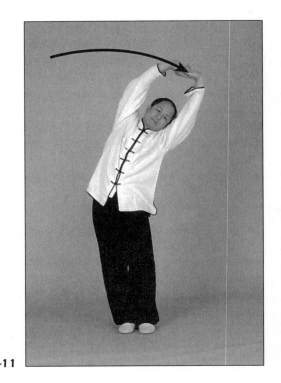

6-10   6-11

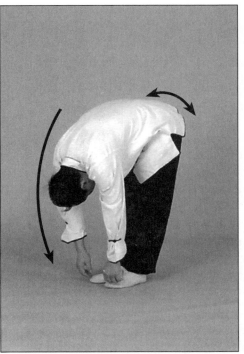

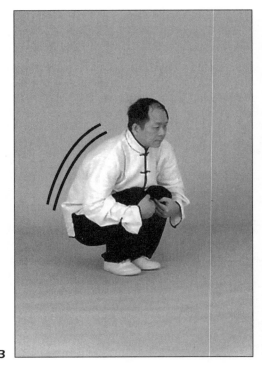

6-12   6-13

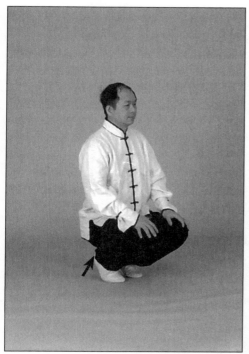 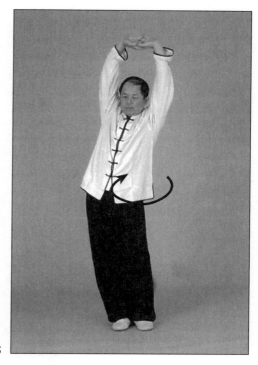

6-14   6-15

muscles/tendons located on the front and the back side of your neck (Figure 6-16). When you stretch your front neck muscles/tendons, you may turn your head backward diagonally while pressing your shoulder backward (Figure 6-17). Start the stretching gently for twenty seconds, then shift the stretching to the rear neck muscles/tendons. When you stretch your rear neck muscles/tendons, simply move your head downward and toward the side (Figure 6-18). Again, stretch for twenty seconds. After you have gone through the four sets of muscles/tendons, repeat from the beginning for another twenty seconds each. You should stretch each muscle/tendon group at least three times. This will provide good stimulation to the muscles/tendons through stretching.

After you have stretched the four neck muscle/tendon groups, extend your head forward with the four muscle/tendon groups evenly stretched (Figure 6-19). To make the stretching more efficient, you may gently push both of your shoulders backward. The goal is to stretch the ligaments instead of the muscles and tendons. Stay in this stretching position for twenty seconds, then turn your head to your left slowly, and then to your right slowly (Figure 6-20). This will help you stretch and loosen up the ligaments in the neck. Repeat the turning two more times on each side.

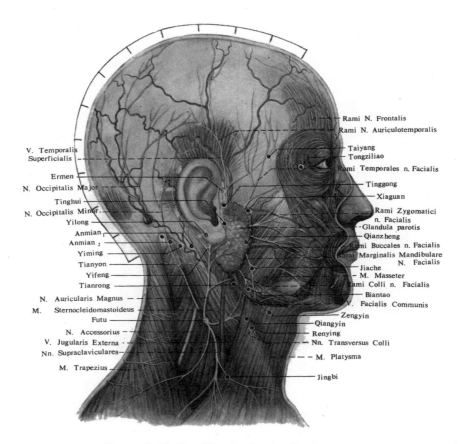

Figure 6-16. The Muscles in the Neck

Finally, gently circle your head to one side about ten times, and then the other side for another ten times (Figure 6-21). You should not circle your neck to its extreme range of motion, since this may damage your cartilage and neck joints. This is a common cause of arthritis in the lower neck area in later life.

Spine Qigong

Next, we will introduce two major Qigong exercises which can heal and rebuild the strength of the back. The first is a set of moving soft and soft-hard Qigong which developed from White Crane and Taijiquan martial styles. It is well known that soft and soft-hard Qigong can be used to improve the Qi and blood circulation, and also to rebuild the strength of the ligaments, tendons and muscles in the back. Therefore, these exercises can be used effectively and efficiently for healing if you already have a back pain problem. In fact, these soft and soft-hard Qigong sets are recommended for those who already have some back pain problems. Generally, if you do these exercises twice per day, you should see some significant improvement in three

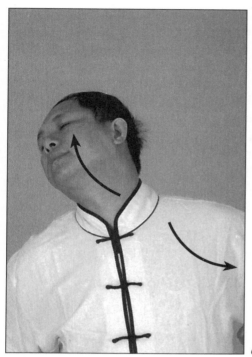

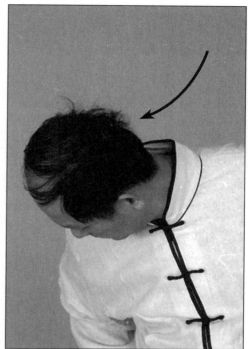

6-17   6-18

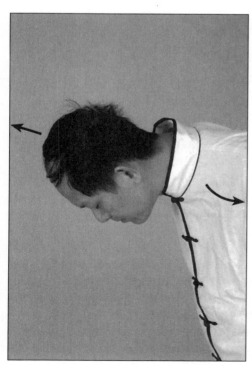

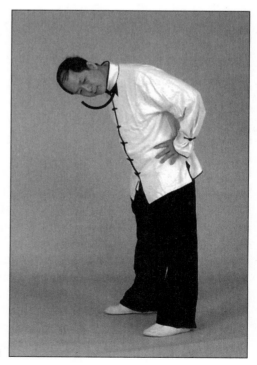

6-19   6-20

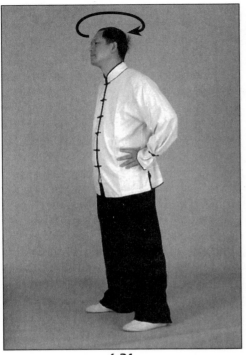

6-21

months, and nearly complete healing in six months. Qigong is not a drug but an exercise to rebuild the strength of your physical body. It takes both time and patience.

The second set is a still hard Qigong which was developed in the Shaolin Temple. The training aims for the reconditioning and rebuilding of the strength and endurance of the muscles and tendons. Once your body has good support from strong torso muscles and tendons, the pressure on the vertebrae joints will be significantly reduced. It is commonly known that when the torso muscles and tendons are weak due to aging or lack of exercise, the pressure on the vertebrae joints will be increased.

From this, you can see that when you do soft and soft-hard spinal Qigong, the exercises can reach deeply, and healing will be more internal. Once you have cured the problem, then you must build up a firm and strong physical torso.

Soft and Soft-Hard Qigong

The torso is supported by the spine and the trunk muscles. Once you have stretched your trunk muscles, you can loosen up the torso. This also moves the muscles inside your body around, which moves and relaxes your internal organs. This, in turn, makes it possible for the Qi to circulate smoothly inside your body. Next, I would like to introduce a few torso movements which I believe are the most beneficial Qigong exercises from my experience.

Once you have mastered all of the movements skillfully, you should learn to bring your mind into a deeper meditative state which allows you to feel and sense the deeper places in your body. Then, through the coordination of the mind, the breathing and the physical movements, lead the Qi to the injured place for healing and lead the accumulated stagnant Qi away from the injured area. We have explained the theory of all of these internal practices in the earlier sections. To make the healing more effective, you need the "unification and harmonization of the internal and external."

1. **Spine Sigh Movement (Jizhuai Tan Xi, 脊椎嘆息).** Spine sigh movement is very important to the back pain patient. This movement imitates the spine's natural action when you sigh. Normally, when you are making a deep sigh, you are sick, sad or depressed. When this happens, your inhalation is longer than exhalation, and the Qi in your torso is more trapped inside, which can therefore cause your torso muscles and spine to become more tense. In addition,

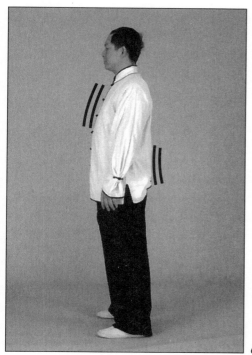 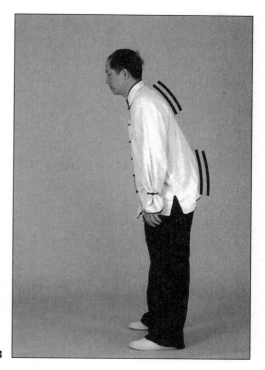

6-22   6-23

the Qi stagnation can also occur in the internal organs and result in sickness. Under these circumstances, instinctively you will inhale deeply while thrusting your chest out, and then push your pelvis out slightly to loosen the lower back (Figure 6-22). Finally, you make the sound of Hen and exhale naturally while continuing to move your spine like a wave upward into the upper body (Figure 6-23). From these repeated sighing movements, the tension of the torso can be eased and the internal organs can be more relaxed.

In order to loosen the lower back when you have pain, you should first be familiar with this spine sigh movement. To practice this movement, place both your arms comfortably in front of your chest. When you inhale, thrust your chest out while straightening up your torso (tailbone pushed forward)(Figure 6-24) and then continue your inhalation while pushing your pelvis backward and gradually holding in your chest (Figure 6-25). When this happens, the Mingmen (Gv-4) cavity on the back will be opened and the Qi in the front and the rear side of the torso will be balanced (Figure 6-26). Finally, release the carbon dioxide and continue pushing the lower back backward to relax it (Figure 6-27). Mingmen is translated as "Life Door" in Chinese medicine, because it is understood that this is the gate which connects with the center of our life, the Real Dan Tian. The Mingmen cavity is located between the 2nd and 3rd lumbar vertebrae. **To release tension in the lower back, the first task is to relax and open this gate by gently and slightly pushing the**

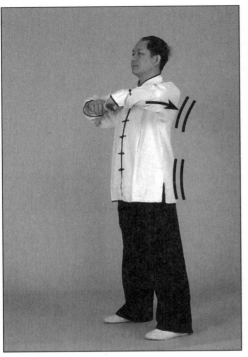 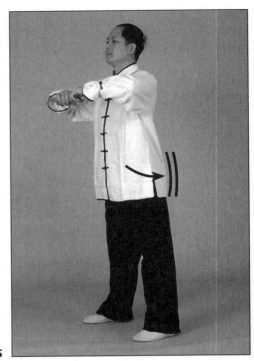

6-24   6-25

pelvis backward. If you have already experienced back pain, you must learn how to move your pelvis correctly to relax the lower back area.

When you do this correctly, you will feel the relaxation so deeply in the spine that it reaches the ligaments of the vertebrae. Remember, whenever you experience lower back pain or tightness, the first step is to repeat this spine sigh movement to loosen up the lower back

2. **Circle the Waist Horizontally (Pin Yuan Niu Yao, 平圓扭腰).** This exercise helps you to regain conscious control of the muscles in your abdomen. The Lower Dan Tian is the main residence of your Original Qi. The Qi in your Lower Dan Tian can be led easily only when your abdomen is loose and relaxed. These abdominal exercises are probably the most important of all the internal Qigong practices.

To practice this exercise, squat down slightly. Without moving your thighs or upper body, use the waist muscles to move the abdomen around in a horizontal circle (Figure 6-28). You should pay attention to the circling of the lower back area. Circle in one direction about ten times and then in the other direction about ten times. If you hold one hand over your Lower Dan Tian and the other on your sacrum, you may be able to focus your attention better on the area you want to control.

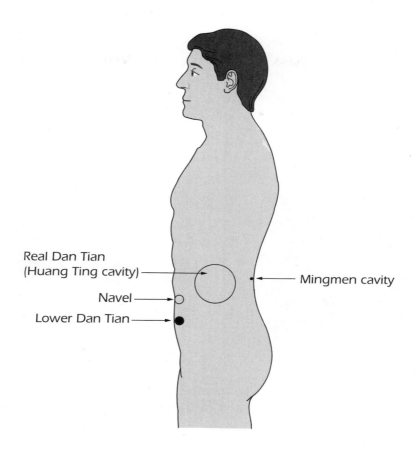

Real Dan Tian
(Huang Ting cavity)

Navel

Lower Dan Tian

Mingmen cavity

Figure 6-26. The Real Dan Tian

In the beginning, you may have difficulty making your body move the way you want. But if you keep practicing, you will quickly learn how to do it. Once you can do the movement comfortably, make the circles larger and larger. Naturally, this will cause the muscles to tense somewhat and inhibit the Qi flow, but the more you practice the sooner you will again be able to relax. After you have practiced for a while and can control your waist muscles easily, start making the circles smaller and also start using your Yi to lead the Qi from the Lower Dan Tian to move in these circles. The final goal is to have only a slight physical movement, but a strong movement of Qi.

There are four major benefits to this abdominal exercise. First, when your Lower Dan Tian area is loose, the Qi can flow in and out easily. This is especially important for health since the Lower Dan Tian is the main source of Qi. Second, when the abdominal area is loose, the Qi circulation in the large and small intestines will be smooth and they can absorb nutrients and eliminate waste. If your body does not eliminate effectively, the absorption of nutrients

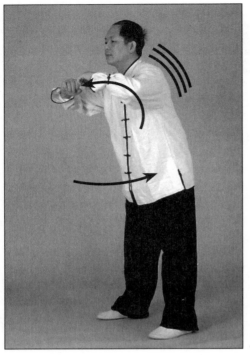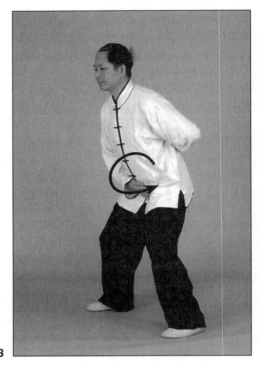

6-27   6-28

will be hindered and you may become sick. Third, when the abdominal area is loose, the Qi in the kidneys will circulate smoothly and the Original Essence stored in the kidneys can be converted more efficiently into Qi. In addition, when the kidney area is loosened, the kidney Qi can be led downward and upward to nourish the entire body. Fourth, these exercises eliminate Qi stagnation in the lower back, healing and preventing lower back pain. Furthermore, this exercise can also help you rebuild the strength of the muscles in the waist area.

If you find that there is too much pain when you stand up to circle the lower back, you may use your hands to support part of the body's weight by leaning against a wall, chair or table (Figure 6-29). The whole idea is to move the lower vertebrae and improve the Qi and blood circulation there. Once you are stronger, you should practice standing and do more repetitions. How many circles you do in each practice depends on your condition. You should proceed cautiously and gradually.

3. **Waving the Spine and Massaging the Internal Organs (Ji Zhui Bo Dong, Nei Zang An Mo, 脊椎波動，內臟按摩).** Beneath your diaphragm is your stomach, on its right is your liver and on its left is your spleen. Once you can comfortably do the movement in your lower abdomen, change the movement from horizontal to vertical and extend it up to your diaphragm. Move your vertebrae joint by joint. What you are aiming for is the movement of the ligaments

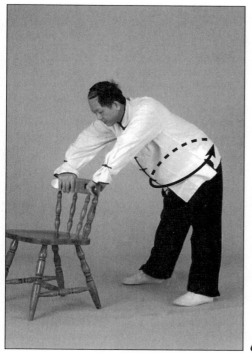 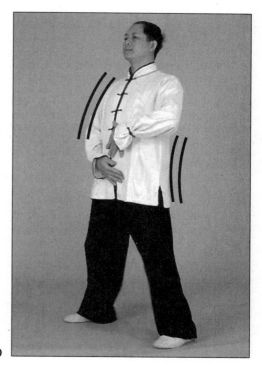

6-29   6-30

which connect the joints. The deep places of the joints must be moved in order to heal.

The easiest way to loosen the area around the diaphragm is to use a wave-like motion between the perineum and the diaphragm (Figures 6-30 to 6-32). You may find it helpful when you practice this to place one hand on your Lower Dan Tian and your other hand above it with the thumb on the solar plexus. Use a forward and backward wave-like motion, flowing up to the diaphragm and down to the perineum and back. Practice ten times.

Next, continue the movement while turning your body slowly to one side and then to the other (Figure 6-33). This will slightly tense the muscles and tendons on one side and loosen them on the other, which will massage the internal organs. The will also gently and gradually stretch and condition the ligaments and rebuild the strength. Repeat ten times on each side.

You may also practice this waving exercise while you are sitting either at a desk or while driving (Figure 6-34). The most important part of this practice is to reach as deep as possible in the movements. In order to reach this goal, your mind must be able to reach deeply, and the movements of the muscles/tendons must be correct. Too tense is not good and too relaxed will not serve any purpose.

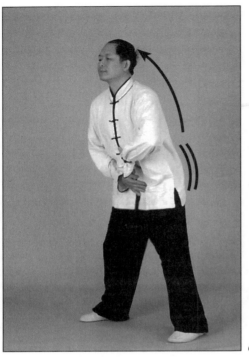
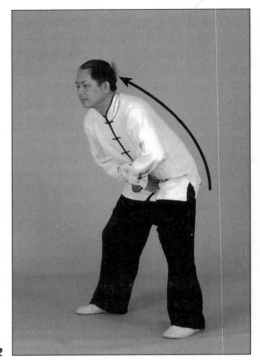

6-31   6-32

4. **Thrust the Chest and Arc the Chest (Tan Xiong Gong Bei, 袒胸拱背).** After
loosening up the center portion of your body, extend the movement up to
your chest and upper spine. The wave-like movement starts in the sacrum
and moves up to the chest. You may find it easier to feel the movement if you
hold one hand on your abdomen and the other lightly on your chest. You
should also coordinate with the shoulders' movement. Inhale when you
move your shoulders backward (Figure 6-35) and exhale when you move
them forward (Figure 6-36). If you remember the sigh movement, you can see
that this is actually a large scale version of the same movement. The inhalation and exhalation should be as deep as possible and the entire chest should
be very loose. When you move your spine, you should be able to feel the vertebrae move section by section. Repeat the motion ten times.

This exercise loosens up the chest and helps to regulate and improve the Qi
circulation in the lungs. Moreover, this kind of wave-like spine movement will
not only improve the Qi and blood circulation at the vertebrae joints for healing, but it will also gradually recondition your spine structure from weak to
strong. Remember, spine movement is the key to maintaining spinal health.
This is also the key to strengthening your immune system.

Again, you may practice this spine movement while sitting as well as standing. Simply generate the wave motion from the sacrum and move it upward
while coordinating with your breathing (Figures 6-37 and 6-38). Be aware of

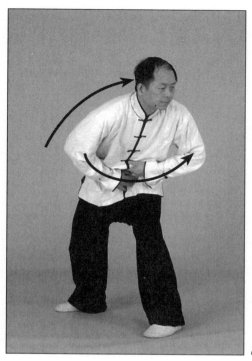

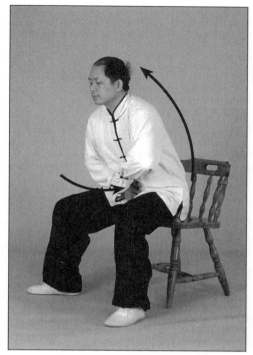

6-33   6-34

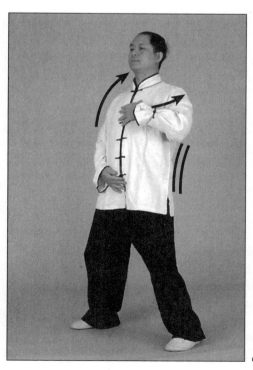

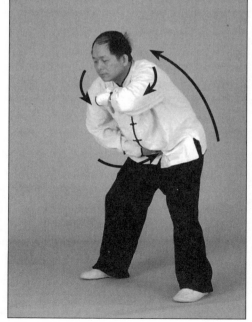

6-35   6-36

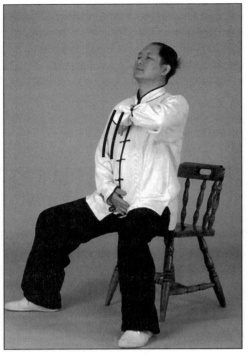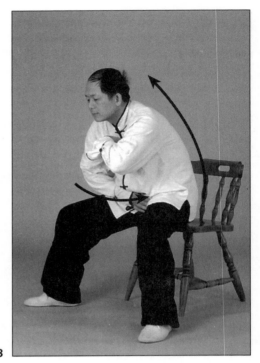

6-37   6-38

the stiffness of your spine whenever you sit for too long while either driving or working. Lift your arms up and stretch your torso first. Then perform the above spinal movements to exercise the spine and loosen it.

5. **White Crane Waves Its Wing (Bai He Dou Chi, 白鶴抖翅).** Once you have completed the loosening up of the chest area and spine, extend the motion to your arms and fingers. When you extend the movement to the arms, you first place your both palms in front of your abdominal area, facing forward. Next, generate the wave motion from the legs or the waist and direct this power upward. It passes through the chest and shoulders and finally reaches the arms (Figures 6-39 to 6-41). Repeat at least ten times. Naturally, if you feel comfortable, you may practice more.

Right after you have finished the above two hands' waving exercises, you should then practice one hand waving exercises. The additional benefit which you may obtain over two hands' waving is you are now twisting your joints from the ankles, hips, spine and finally reaching to the finger tips. Do not twist your knees. This will help to loosen and strengthen the joint areas. When you practice with one arm, again you place both your palms right in front of your abdominal area with the right palm facing out and the left palm lightly touching the abdomen (Figure 6-42). Then, you generate the twisting motion from the bottom of your feet, upward through the knees and hips, through every section of the spine, and finally allowing it to pass through the

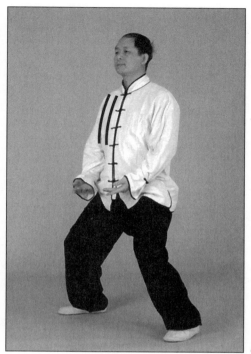

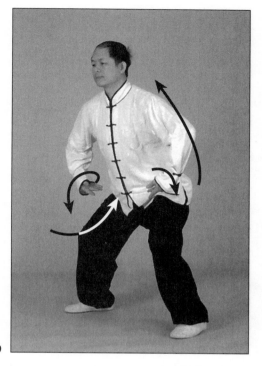

6-39   6-40

shoulders and reach to the finger tips (Figures 6-43 and 6-44). Practice ten time for each arm..

Again, you may practice this Qigong exercise while you are sitting (Figures 6-45 to 6-48). These exercises will loosen up every joint in your body from the waist to the fingers. Moreover, they lead the Qi out from the central body to the limbs. If you are not leading the excess Qi out, the body will become too Yang and you may become tense again. The key to healing and relaxation is to lead the excess Qi out of the body through the limbs. These movements have been found beneficial for healing chest problems such as asthma, chest cancer, lung problems and heart problems.

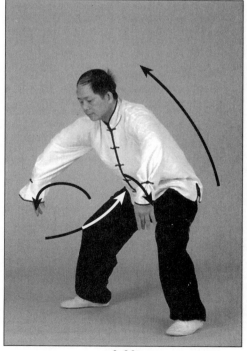

6-41

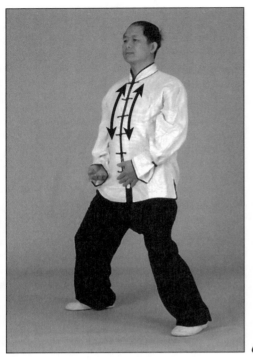
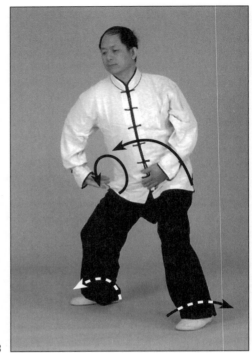

6-42   6-43

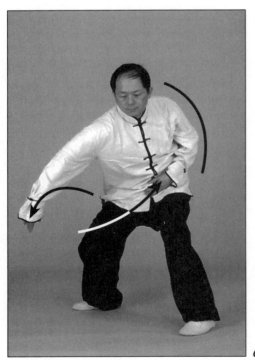
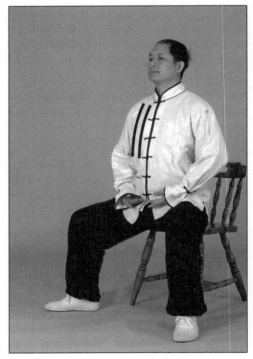

6-44   6-45

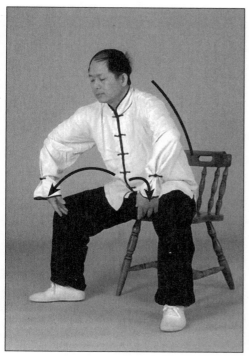

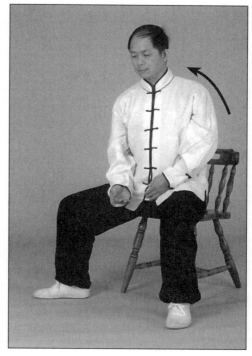

6-46   6-47

6. Recovery. After you have completed the above spine waving movements, continue to lead the Qi out of your body through the limbs. The easiest way is to swing your arms forward and backward by imitating a natural human activity—walking. Simply swing your arms forward to the height of the shoulders (Figure 6-49) and then let them drop and swing back by themselves (Figure 6-50). Repeat about two hundred times. Naturally, you may swing from five minutes to half an hour depending on your health. Swinging the arms is one of the easiest laymen Qigong practices, simple and easy for anyone.

Next, continue your swinging while at the same time walking in place

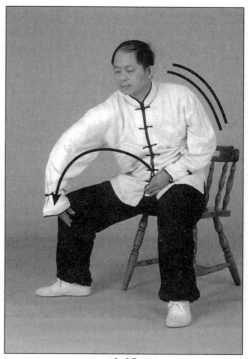

6-48

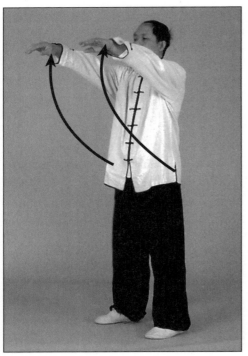 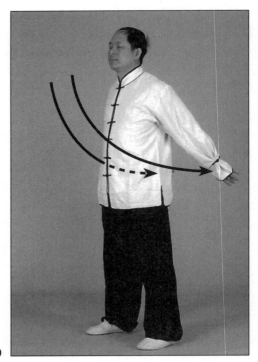

6-49   6-50

with your knees as high as your hips. Every time you raise your knee, you gently push back your lower back (Figure 6-51). This will generate a comfortable forward and backward movement to exercise the lower back. Again if it is comfortable start with fifty steps and when you feel stronger, increase the number of repetitions.

Finally, you should lead the Qi to the bottom of your feet. Continue your arm swinging. When your arms are lifting, raise your heels and when your arms are down, make your heels touch the floor (Figure 6-52). Repeat about twenty to thirty times. If you start with more than thirty, you may experience cramping in your calf.

When you practice this exercise, you do not have to worry about your breathing. Simply breathe naturally and smoothly. You may even watch television while your are swinging your arms. This is why it is called laymen Qigong. It is simple and easy, without too much training of concentrated mind and breathing.

Still Hard Qigong

As mentioned earlier, still hard Qigong focuses on building the strength and endurance of the muscles and tendons. However, **the training will contribute only slightly to the ligaments' reconditioning**. The reason for this is simply that in order to build up the muscles and tendons and reach a healthy level, the muscles and tendons must be tensed up during the training. When this happens, the joints will be more tense and locked. This will therefore limit the mobility of the joint movements and the ligaments will not be conditioned.

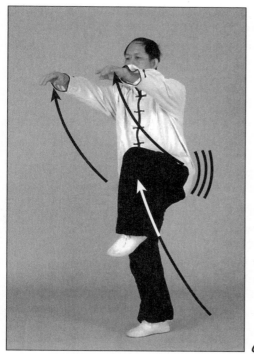
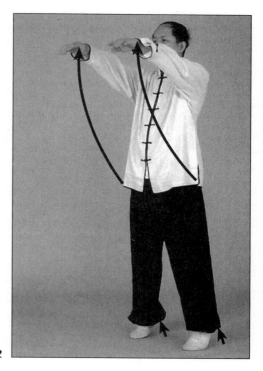

6-51   6-52

1. **Taiji Arcing Arms (Taiji Gong Shou, 太極拱手).** Taiji arcing arms is a Taiji training which specializes in conditioning the strength and endurance of the torso and spine, especially the lower back area. It is a standing still meditation. This training is not as hard and tense as that of the Shaolin training called Iron Board Bridge, which will be introduced next. Therefore, if you have treated your spine problem, you may want to strengthen your torso and gradually increase its endurance. This is the way to prevent back pain from happening again.

When you train, stand with one leg solidly on the ground while the other foot gently touches the floor by its toes. In addition, raise both your arms to shoulder height with your palms facing your chest (Figure 6-53). When you do this, if your left leg is touching by its toes, your right side back muscles and tendons will be more tensed than the left side. You should stand in this position for three minutes at the beginning and then switch your legs for another three minutes without moving your arms. This will condition the left side of back muscles and tendons. When you practice, breathe naturally and smoothly. If possible, keep your mind aware internally to feel the training, especially the torso's condition.

After you practice for a while and feel your torso getting stronger, then you may increase the time you stand. In Taijiquan practice, often a practitioner will stand for fifteen to thirty minutes on each leg. Even though this training

171

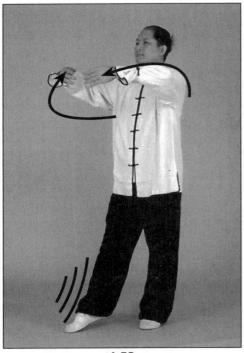

6-53

builds up strength and endurance slowly and gradually, there is no risk involved. It is recommended for those people who have a weak torso and spine.

2.   Iron Board Bridge (Tie Ban Qiao, 鐵板橋). Iron Board Bridge is well known in the external styles of Chinese martial arts. The main purpose of the training is to build a stronger and more durable torso for power manifestation and also to prevent injury to the spine.

In this training, at the beginning, simply lie on your back and lift your head and heels a couple of inches off the ground (Figure 6-54). Both legs should be straight. The distance from your head to the ground and also from the heels to the ground should not be too high. If they are too high, pressure will build up in the lower spine and generate injury. A proper height for the lifting of the head and the heels can keep the rear side of the torso stretched and the front side properly tensed.

You should at between thirty seconds and one minute. After you have trained for some time, if you feel comfortable, increase to two minutes and so on until you can hold it for three minutes. If you can reach this goal, you have built up a very good level of strength in your torso.

When you train, you should take your time. Do not hold your breath while training. Hasty training can only harm you. You should remember that **your body must be conditioned slowly and gradually**. If you have too much ego, once you have injured yourself, it will take a long time to heal, and if you have injured yourself once, you will never be quite the same. The results of mistraining can be devastating.

The above Qigong practices have been experienced for hundreds and some for a thousand years, and they have proven very effective and beneficial for spinal healing and strength rebuilding. You should build up your confidence and proceed with healing and reconditioning slowly and gradually. **Always pay attention to your body, feel it and communicate with it**. Moreover, you should also analyze and understand the conditions and the theory of the practice. Once you have built up a firm and solid theoretical and practical root, you may find other postures or movements which can help your healing and reconditioning to proceed faster and more suitably for you.

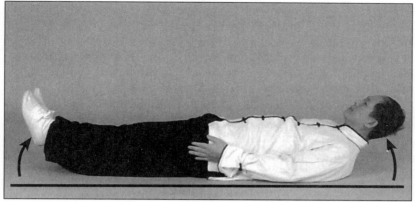

6-54

6-4. Massage for Back Pain

Using massage to alleviate back pain includes two parts. The first part is to use the general massage techniques such as Pushing (Tui, 推), Grabbing (Na, 拿), Rubbing (Rou, 揉), etc. to massage the back. There are a few specific purposes associated with general massage:

1. To relax the muscles/tendons.
2. To improve the blood and Qi circulation.
3. To ease pain and feel more comfortable both physically and mentally.

The second part is, during general massage treatments, you may also apply pressure to some specific acupuncture cavities. This is commonly called Cavity Press (Dian Xue, 點穴) or acupressure. Again, the purposes of using cavity press are:

1. Like acupuncture, to anesthetize the local area to alleviate or stop pain.
2. To bring accumulated Qi or blood hidden deeply in the body to the surface.
3. To improve the Qi and blood circulation.

You should know that the main goal of massage is to ease pain and make the patient feel more comfortable. However, often after massage treatment, the patient will experience soreness or even some pain. According to Chinese massage theory, these phenomena are quite normal. The reason for this is that after massage, the Qi and blood circulation is improved and this enlivens the sensitivity of the nerves around the massaged area. If you experience this, simply move the sore area for a few minutes, and the soreness will gradually fade.

At this point, you should understand that though massage is able to expedite the healing process and temporarily cure the symptoms, as long as your physical body is weak, back pain will return. Therefore, whenever you feel comfortable, you should do Qigong exercises to strengthen the structure of your physical body. This is the way of curing the problem at its root. If you are interested in knowing more about Qigong massage, you may refer to the book, *Chinese Qigong Massage*, from YMAA Publication Center.

In this section, we will first introduce the cavities which are commonly used in acupressure and acupuncture for back pain. After you become familiar with these cavities, we will discuss how you can massage yourself when you have back pain. Finally, massage techniques which you may use to help back pain in a patient will be reviewed. Again, you should always keep in your mind that the best way to alleviate pain and promote healing from the root is to encourage your patient to learn and practice the Qigong movements discussed in the last section.

Massaging Cavities for Back Pain

1. **Jianjing (GB-21, 肩井).** Massaging the Jianjing cavity can ease mental tension. Jianjing means "Shoulder Well," and it is the passageway between the neck and the arms (Figure 6-55). Stimulating the Jianjing cavity correctly will not only open up the Qi channels from the head to the arms, but also stimulate the skin and open all the pores. Stimulating this cavity causes a very pleasant, exciting feeling in the patient, and sometimes gives them goose bumps all over the body. Jianjing is frequently used in acupuncture and Qigong to lead the Qi which has accumulated in the head to the arms, thereby relieving headaches and releasing pressure in the head. Normally, when you are in pain, your mind is tense and pressure is built up in your head. Consequently, your physical body is tensed. Massaging the Jianjing cavity can help you release all of this tension.

2. **Shenshu (B-23, 腎俞).** Shenshu means "Two Kidney's Admittance" or "Kidney's Hollow" (Figure 6-55). These two cavities are the immediate entrance and exit of the kidney's Qi to the outside through the back. According to Chinese medical experience, if the kidney's Qi is either too Yang or too Yin, the kidneys will be tensed, which results in tension in the lower back area. In order to regulate the Qi condition in your kidneys, normally whenever the kidney's Qi is too Yang, the excess Qi will be released from these two doors. If the kidneys are too Yin, they may be nourished through these two doors either by acupuncture or massage. From this, you can see that these two doors are used to regulate the Qi conditions in the kidneys.

In order to alleviate pain in your back, you should first release the tension or the pressure in your kidneys. When the kidney are relaxed, the lower back will be relaxed and you will feel comfortable.

There are two other doors or gates on the bottom of feet called "Yongquan." They are also used to regulate the kidney's Qi status. We will discuss the Yongquan cavities later.

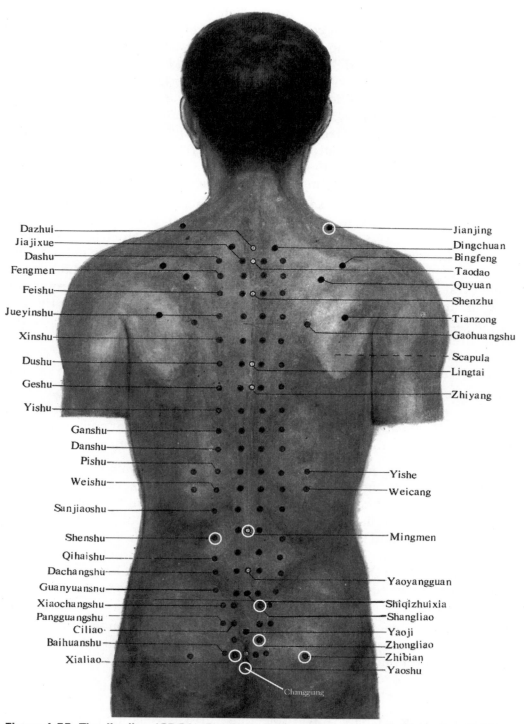

Dazhui
Jiajixue
Dashu
Fengmen
Feishu
Jueyinshu
Xinshu
Dushu
Geshu
Yishu
Ganshu
Danshu
Pishu
Weishu
Sanjiaoshu
Shenshu
Qihaishu
Dachangshu
Guanyuanshu
Xiaochangshu
Pangguangshu
Ciliao
Baihuanshu
Xialiao

Jianjing
Dingchuan
Bingfeng
Taodao
Quyuan
Shenzhu
Tianzong
Gaohuangshu
Scapula
Lingtai
Zhiyang
Yishe
Weicang
Mingmen
Yaoyangguan
Shiqizhuixia
Shangliao
Yaoji
Zhongliao
Zhibian
Yaoshu

Changqiang

Figure 6-55. The Jianjing (GB-21), Shenshu (B-23), Mingmen (Gv-4), Shangliao (B-31), Ciliao (B-32), Zhongliao (B-33), Xialiao (B-34), Zhibian (B-49), and Changqiang (Gv-1) Cavities

3. **Mingmen (Gv-4, 命門).** Mingmen means "Life's Door." It is called this because it is the gate through which you can reach the residence of the Qi: the Lower Dan Tian (Figure 6-55). The Mingmen cavity is located between the spinous processes of the 2nd and 3rd lumbar vertebrae. In Qigong theory, the Lower Dan Tian in your lower abdomen is called "Jia Dan Tian, 假丹田 " which means the "false Dan Tian," while the space between the false Dan Tian and the Mingmen is called "Zhen Dan Tian, 眞丹田 " or the "real Dan Tian" (Figure 6-56). While the false Dan Tian is the furnace which generates Qi, the real Dan Tian is the residence (or battery) which stores the Qi which has been generated. According to Chinese medicine, Qi is the origin of life. The Mingmen is therefore the door to reach this Qi storage place.

4. **Baliao (B-31-34, 八髎 i.e., sacrum).** Baliao includes eight cavities on the sacrum, four on each side. These include Shangliao (B-31, 上髎), Ciliao (B-32, 次髎), Zhongliao (B-33, 中髎), and Xialiao (B-34, 下髎)(Figure 6-55). In Chinese Qigong, the sacrum is the junction where the Qi enters the spinal cord and reaches up to the brain. The sacrum is called "Xian Gu" (仙骨), which means "immortal bone." This is because, from correct Qigong training through the sacrum area in advanced Qigong practice, a practitioner can reach the goal of Buddhahood or enlightenment and then immortality. In order to reach this goal, the Qi must be led upward through the Thrusting Vessel (Chong Mai, 衝脈) in the spinal cord to reach the brain and nourish the spirit. To do this, you need to learn how to lead the Qi into the spinal cord through the sacrum.

    Massaging the sacrum, in addition to sending a pleasant sensation to the brain, also sends Qi from the back to the bottom of the feet. Consequently, the lower back can be relaxed. This is because the sacrum connects the Qi from the legs with the Qi that goes all the way to the brain.

5. **Changqiang (Gv-1, 長強).** Changqiang (Long Strength) is also called "Weilu," which means "tailbone." The Changqiang cavity is the first cavity on the Yang Governing Vessel where the Qi circulation leaves the Yin Conception Vessel (Figure 6-55). It is believed in Chinese Qigong that, as you get older, this cavity seals up more and more, which interferes with normal Qi circulation in the Governing and Conception Vessels. When this happens, the Qi circulating in the twelve primary Qi channels will be affected and the Qi level in the twelve internal organs will not be regulated smoothly. It is believed that this is the cause of aging.

    When you massage this tailbone, through comfortable stimulation, you will lead the Qi downward to the end of the spinal cord. This will soothe the tension in the lower back area caused by pain. The tailbone is just one of the two ends of a piece of rope. From the stimulation of one end, the Qi stagnating in the rope can be led to the other end.

6. **Huiyin (Co-1, 會陰).** The Huiyin (Meeting Yin) cavity is located in the perineum, midway between the genitals and the anus (Figure 6-57). In Chinese

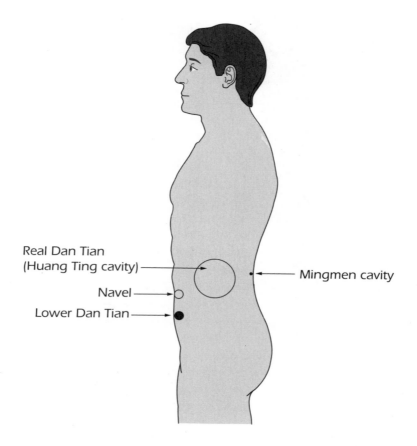

Real Dan Tian
(Huang Ting cavity)

Navel

Lower Dan Tian

Mingmen cavity

Figure 6-56. The Real Dan Tian

medicine and Qigong, the Huiyin is considered one of the most important cavities. It is the junction of many vessels, including the Conception (Ren Mai, 任脈), Governing (Du Mai, 督脈), Thrusting (Chong Mai, 衝脈), Yin Heel (Yinchiao Mai, 陰蹻脈), and Yin Linking (Yinwei Mai, 陰維脈) Vessels. Remember, according to Chinese medicine, vessels are like reservoirs which regulate the Qi circulating in the twelve primary Qi channels.

When you massage this cavity, the Qi will be led farther down to the bottom of body which makes it easier to lead it to the legs. Naturally, if massaging this cavity will cause your patient tension and uneasiness, you should skip this cavity.

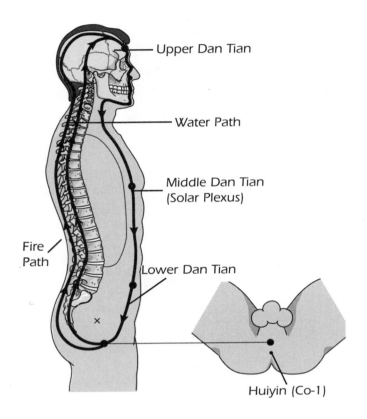

- Upper Dan Tian
- Water Path
- Middle Dan Tian (Solar Plexus)
- Fire Path
- Lower Dan Tian
- Huiyin (Co-1)

Figure 6-57. The Huiyin Cavity (Co-1)

7. **Juliao (GB-29, 居髎), Zhibian (B-49, 秩邊), and Huantiao (GB-30, 環跳).** Juliao means "Stationary Seam," Zhibian means "Order's Edge," and Huantiao means "Encircling Leap" (Figures 6-55 and 6-58). The hip is considered to be the junction of the Qi and blood exchange between the legs and the body. When these three cavities are stimulated, the Qi accumulated in the lower back can be led downward and to the side of the hip. If you pay attention, you can see that all of these three cavities are also located on the nerves which connect the lower back to the legs. Stimulating these three cavities properly can generate a strong sensation which moves from the lower back to the feet, consequently, the tension of the lower back can be immediately reduced. Frequently, stimulating any of these three cavities will also cause the Weizhong cavity on the back of the knee or the Yongquan cavity on the bottom of the foot to also be stimulated. This multiple stimulation leads the Qi straight down to the knee or to the bottom of the feet. We will discuss the Weizhong and Yongquan cavities later.

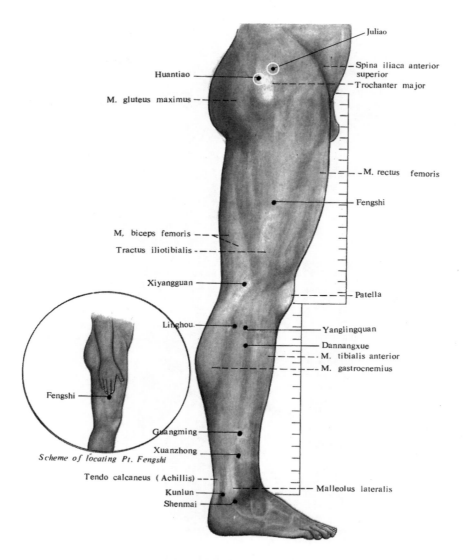

Figure 6-58. The Juliao (GB-29) and Huantiao (GB-30) Cavities

8. **Chengfu (B-50, 承扶), Weizhong (B-54, 委中), and Chengshan (B-57, 承山).** Chengfu means "Receive Support," Weizhong means "Commission the Middle" and Chengshan means "Support the Mountain." These three cavities are also on the path of the sciatic nerve (Figure 6-59). When these three cavities are stimulated, the Qi can be led quickly to the thigh, knee and calf. According to Chinese medical theory, the farther the Qi is led away from the pained area, the more the pain and tension can be reduced.

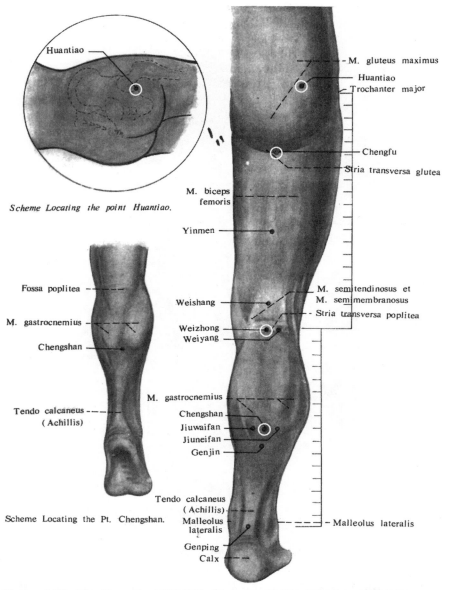

Scheme Locating the point Huantiao.

Scheme Locating the Pt. Chengshan.

Figure 6-59. The Huantiao (GB-30), Chengfu (B-50), Weizhong (B-54), and Chengshan (B-57) Cavities

9. **Yanglingquan (GB-34, 陽陵泉) and Zusanli (S-36, 足三里).** Yanglingquan means "Yang Tomb Spring" and Zusanli means "Three Miles on the Leg" (Figures 6-60 and 6-61). When these two cavities are massaged and stimulated, the Qi can be led continuously to the calf.

10. **Jiexi (S-41, 解溪) and Yongquan (K-1, 湧泉).** Jiexi (Release Stream) is located in the middle of the crease in the front of the ankle (Figure 6-62). When Jiexi is pressed and stimulated, the Qi on the front of the thigh can be led downward.

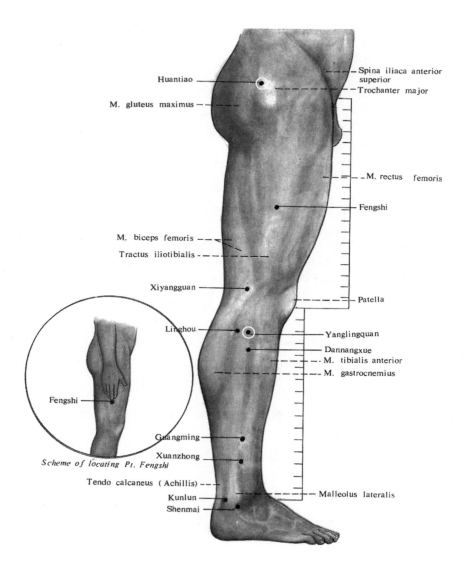

Spina iliaca anterior
superior

Trochanter major

Huantiao

M. gluteus maximus

M. rectus femoris

Fengshi

M. biceps femoris

Tractus iliotibialis

Xiyangguan

Patella

Linghou

Yanglingquan

Dannangxue

M. tibialis anterior

M. gastrocnemius

Fengshi

Scheme of locating Pt. Fengshi

Guangming

Xuanzhong

Tendo calcaneus (Achillis)

Malleolus lateralis

Kunlun

Shenmai

Figure 6-60. The Huantiao (GB-30) and Yanglingquan (GB-34) Cavities

Yongquan is commonly translated as "Bubbling Well" or "Gushing Spring" (Figure 6-63). This cavity is located on the sole of the foot, one third of the way from the base of the second toe to the heel. This cavity is an important Qi gate which regulates the Qi in the kidneys. Stimulating this cavity will lead Qi from the torso downward to the bottom of the feet and spread it out there.

11. Other Local Non-Acupuncture Cavities. When you have back pain, there are some areas which are especially sore or aching. You may gently massage

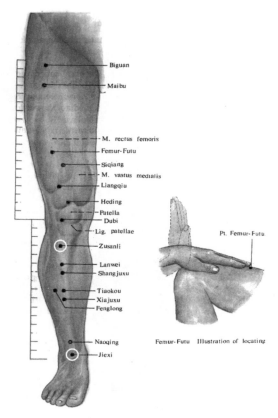

Figure 6-61. The Zusanli (S-36) and Jiexi (S-41) Cavities

these areas to spread the Qi and blood accumulation away from the areas and improve circulation.

General Massage Rules

1. **From center to sides.** This is to spread the Qi and blood accumulation or stagnation from the center of the body to the sides. This will loosen the tightness of the muscles and tendons at the central spinal area (Figure 6-64). This also leads the stagnant Qi to the arms. When this rule is applied to lower back pain, the Qi stagnation in the lower back is led to the sides and also to the arms.

2. **From top to bottom.** Generally, the purpose of this is to lead the accumulated or stagnant Qi downward to the legs (Figure 6-64). When this rule is applied to lower back pain, the Qi is led from the lower back to the bottoms of the feet.

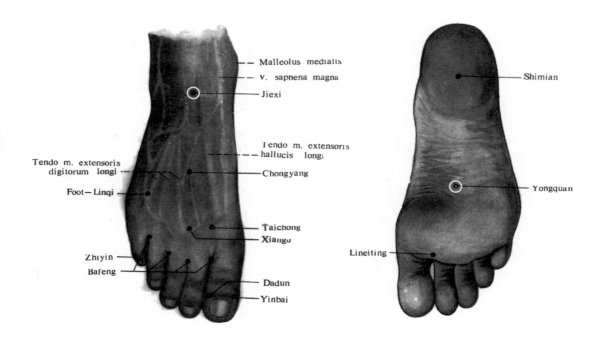

Malleolus medialis
v. saphena magna
Jiexi
Tendo m. extensoris hallucis longi
Tendo m. extensoris digitorum longi
Foot—Linqi
Chongyang
Taichong
Xiangu
Zhiyin
Bafeng
Dadun
Yinbai

Shimian
Yongquan
Lineiting

Figure 6-62. The Jiexi (S-41) Cavity   **Figure 6-63. The Yongquan (K-1)**

3. **From shallow to deep and then from deep to shallow.** First, you loosen the tension of the muscles by shallow massage. Shallow gentle massage on the muscles can make your patient relax and feel easy and comfortable. When your patient is relaxed, then you can reach deep with acupressure techniques and bring the Qi and blood stagnation to the surface. If you are not able to reach deep places in the joints, then the Qi and blood accumulation and stagnation will remain, and the effectiveness of the massage will be shallow. Finally, right after deep acupressure massage, you should apply shallow massage again to spread the Qi and blood away from the pain area.

General Massage Hand Forms

Before you massage yourself or someone else, you should be familiar with some of the basic techniques, such as which parts of your hands you may use for massage and how it can be done. If you do this correctly, the treatment can be effective.

1. **Base of the palm.** The base of the palm is the most common place you may use to massage someone. Generally, it covers a bigger massage area and is commonly used to loosen up the muscles and tendons. It is not easy if you

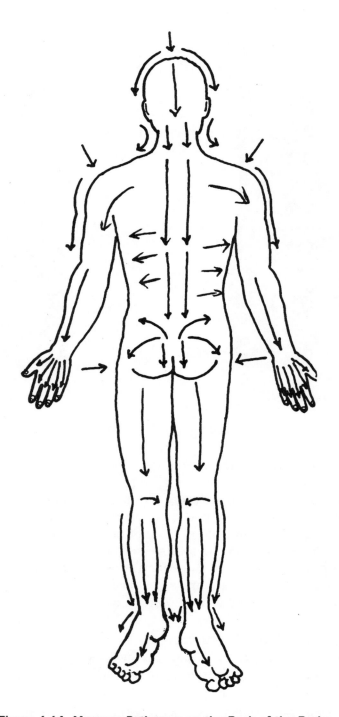

Figure 6-64. Massage Pathways on the Back of the Body

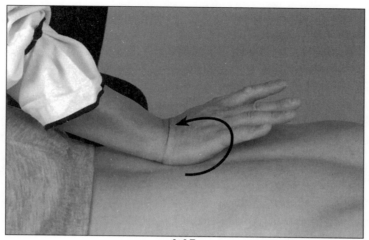

6-65

try to use this place to massage your own back simply because in order to do so, you must twist your own arms, which does not allow for good leverage to generate power. However, this technique can be used to massage someone else effectively. When you use this place to massage someone, you may simply press down with appropriate power to the area needed to be massaged, and then rub with a circular motion (Figure 6-65). **This circular motion should originate from your shoulder and elbow**. Moreover, you should not rub the skin. Instead your palm and skin should stick together and allow the power to reach deep into the muscles. Often, if you need stronger pressing power, you may use both palms for massage (Figure 6-66).

2. **Edge of the palm.** The edge of the palm is the second most common place that you may use to massage someone. Again, it covers a bigger massage area and is commonly used to loosen up the muscles and tendons such as the back muscles. Similarly, this technique is not easy to apply on yourself. When you use this place to massage someone else, you may simply press down with appropriate power to the area to be massaged, and then rub with a circular motion (Figure 6-67). Again, the circular motion should originate from your shoulder and elbow. Moreover, you should not rub the skin. Instead your palm and skin should stick together to allow the power reach deep into the muscles. If you need more pressing power, you may press your other hand on the top of the wrist area of the massaging hand (Figure 6-68).

3. **Thumb and index finger.** The thumb and index fingers are specially used for cavity acupressure simply because they can generate deep penetrating power into a tiny place. When the thumb is used, the index finger is used to support the strength of the thumb's pressing (Figure 6-69). However, when the index finger is used for acupressure, often either the thumb is used to support the strength (Figure 6-70) or both the thumb and middle finger are

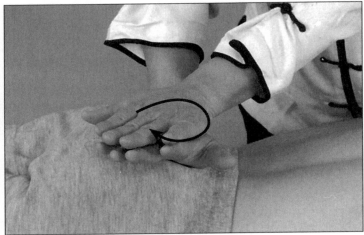

6-66

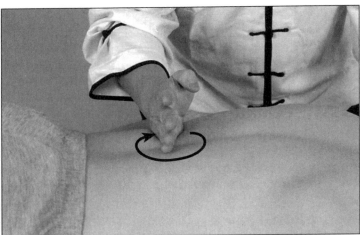

6-67

used together (Figure 6-71). When the thumb or index finger is used for acupressure, the finger is firmly pressed in and then vibrations are generated from the wrist and the forearm for stimulation (Figure 6-72).

4. **Base knuckle of the pinkie.** If you use the base knuckle to massage, the power can penetrate deeply. Often, the base knuckle is used to press and rub a cavity or specific pain spots. Again, this technique cannot be used to massage your own back easily. When you use this technique to massage someone, simply place the base knuckle of your pinkie on the spot, then press and rub (Figure 6-73). Again, the pressing power and circular rubbing should be generated from your shoulder and elbow.

5. **Middle knuckle of the thumb.** The middle knuckle of the thumb is commonly used to massage the side of the body either for self massage or to massage a partner. When you use this place to massage, you press the tip of your

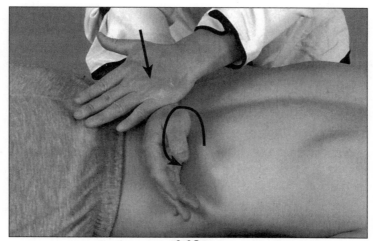

6-68

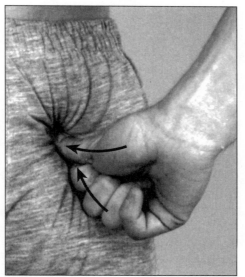

6-69

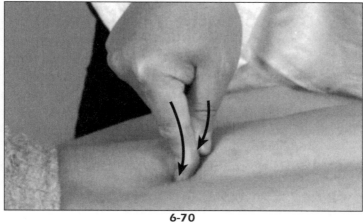

6-70

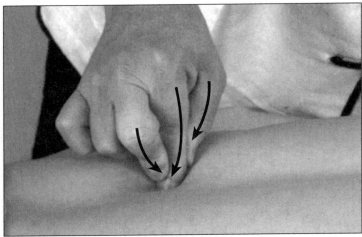

6-71

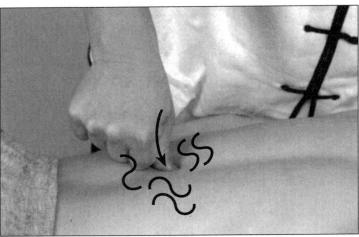

6-72

thumb to the middle section of your index finger to generate support and leverage. Then, press the middle knuckle of the thumb on the spot to be stimulated, and rub with a circular motion (Figure 6-74). Because the power generated from this technique can reach deeply, it is commonly used to massage.

6. **Base knuckle of the index finger.** The base knuckle of your index finger can especially be used for back massage. The leverage is right and the power can be applied very easily. When you do this, simply place your fist on your back and place the base knuckle of your index finger on the spot to be massaged, and then press and rub (Figure 6-75). If you do not want the massage power to penetrate, you may use the side of your fist on the thumb side to massage (Figure 6-76). In this case, the power will be more shallow and you will be more relaxed.

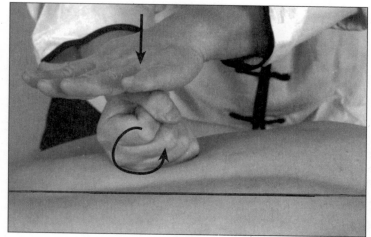

6-73

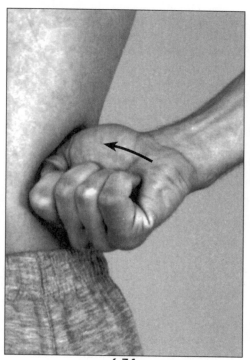

6-74

7. **Forearm.** The forearm is commonly used to massage the big muscles of your partner. It is not easy to use it to massage your own back. When the forearm is used to massage the back muscles, since the power is not penetrating, it can generate a good level of relaxation in your partner. When you use the forearm to massage, simply place your forearm on the muscles to be massaged, using the other hand to press the forearm to generate downward pressure. Then circle your arm using the elbow and shoulder (Figure 6-77).

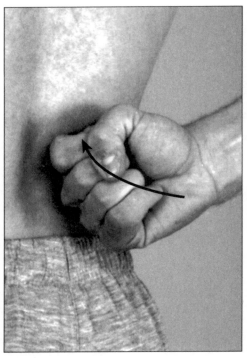 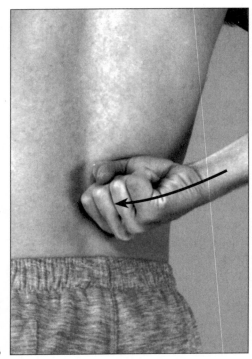

6-75   6-76

Here, we only introduce a few simple but effective hand forms and techniques of massage for back pain. The more you practice, the more proficient you will become. If you keep your mind open, ponder and practice, you may discover many ways of effective massage by yourself. If you would like to know more about Qigong massage techniques, please refer to the book and videotape: *Chinese Qigong Massage*, from YMAA Publication Center.

Self-Massage

It is not easy to massage yourself if you have back pain. The reason for this is that it is not easy for your hands to reach your back and rub it without generating tension in your torso either from twisting or from the pressing of the hands. Therefore, the best way to release the pain is to actually move your lower torso gently and slowly to improve the Qi and blood circulation.

However, often you will discover that through simple hitting or pressing, you can alleviate pain and also help to lead the Qi downward to the bottom of your feet. If you can do this without causing more pain or too much tension in your lower back, then you may effectively soothe the Qi and blood circulation in your back and serve the purpose. As a matter of fact, it is advised that moving and massage techniques be used together. This is the most effective and efficient way. Next, we will introduce the procedures for this combination.

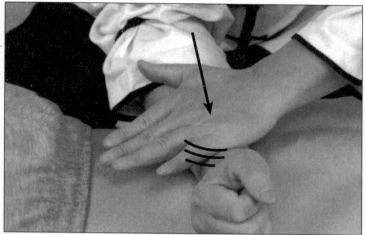

6-77

Step #1. Gently circle your waist area horizontally at least ten times each direction (Figure 6-78). If the pain is serious, make the circle smaller and if the pain is minor, make the circle bigger. The idea is to loosen the muscles and tendons in the waist area. When the tension of this area is reduced and the muscles are more relaxed, the Qi and blood circulation will improve.

Step #2. Bow your torso forward gently to stretch the back muscles and tendons to loosen the tightness of the back caused from the pain (Figure 6-79). How low you bow depends on the level of your pain. If the pain is minor, you may bow lower than that if you have serious pain. You may reach the same goal if you are sitting (Figure 6-80).

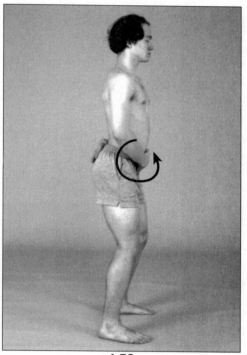

6-78

Next, turn your upper body to the side and gently bow in both directions (Figure 6-81). This will stretch the back muscles more deeply and unlock the tension. Naturally, you may also reach the same goal by sitting down (Figure 6-82).

Step #3. Gently press and rub the muscles of the lower back with the back of your fist (Figure 6-83) or the base knuckle of your index finger (Figure 6-84). This will continue to loosen the muscles of the lower back area.

Step #4. Use the back of your fist to gently hit the Shenshu (B-23, 腎俞), Mingmen

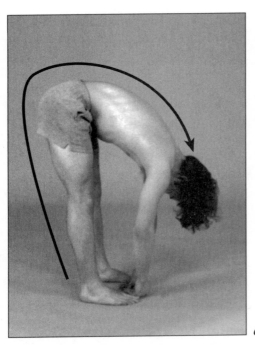 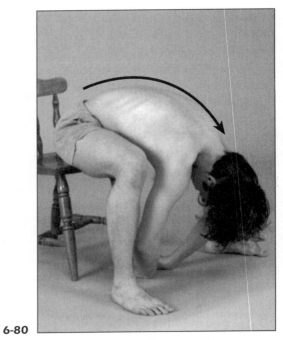

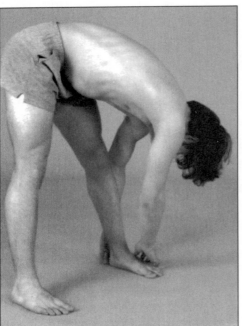 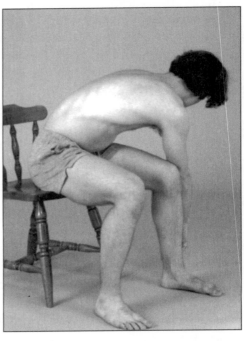

6-79   6-80

6-81   6-82

(Gv-4, 命門), and Baliao (B-31-34, 八髎) cavities (i.e., sacrum)(Figure 6-85).
You should follow the order from the top to the bottom and do not reverse
the order. You may repeat the same process many times until these areas are
comfortably stimulated.

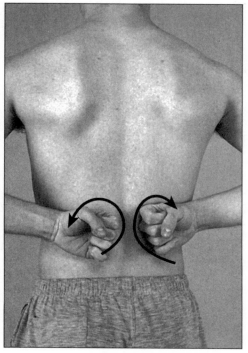 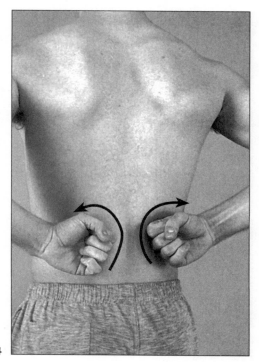

6-83   6-84

Next, use the base knuckle of your index finger to press and rub with circular motion on these cavities (Figure 6-86). Again, follow the order. This effort will make the stimulation reach deeper and help to greatly reduce the pain.

Step #5. Use the base knuckle of your index finger or fist to hit the Zhibian (B-49, 秩邊), Juliao (GB-29, 居髎), and Huantiao (GB-30, 環跳) cavities (Figure 6-87). Again, the purpose is to stimulate these three cavities so the Qi accumulated in the lower back can be led downward.

Next, use the middle knuckle of your thumb or the base knuckle of your index finger to press and rub the same three cavities (Figure 6-88).

Step #6. Use the thumb or index and middle fingers to press and rub the Weizhong (B-54, 委中)(Figure 6-89) and Chengshan cavities (B-57, 承山) (Figure 6-90) for a few times. Then, use the thumb or index finger to press and rub the Yanglingquan (GB-34, 陽陵泉)(Figure 6-91) and Zusanli cavities (S-36, 足三里)(Figure 6-92). Finally, use the thumb to press and rub the Jiexi (S-41, 解溪)(Figure 6-93) and Yongquan (K-1, 湧泉) cavities (Figure 6-94). You may repeat the same process several times. Remember when you stimulate these cavities, start from the top and then downward to the feet. Do not reverse the order.

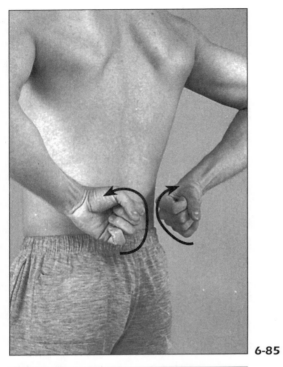

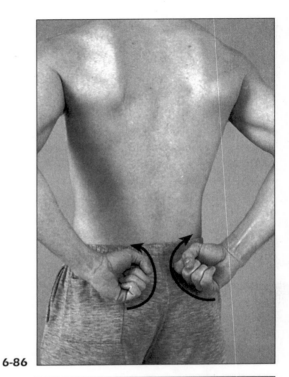

6-85   6-86

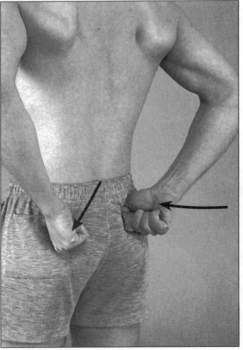

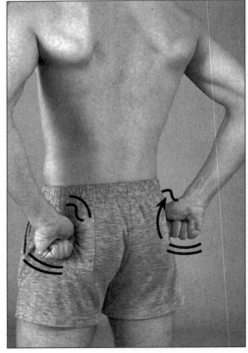

6-87   6-88

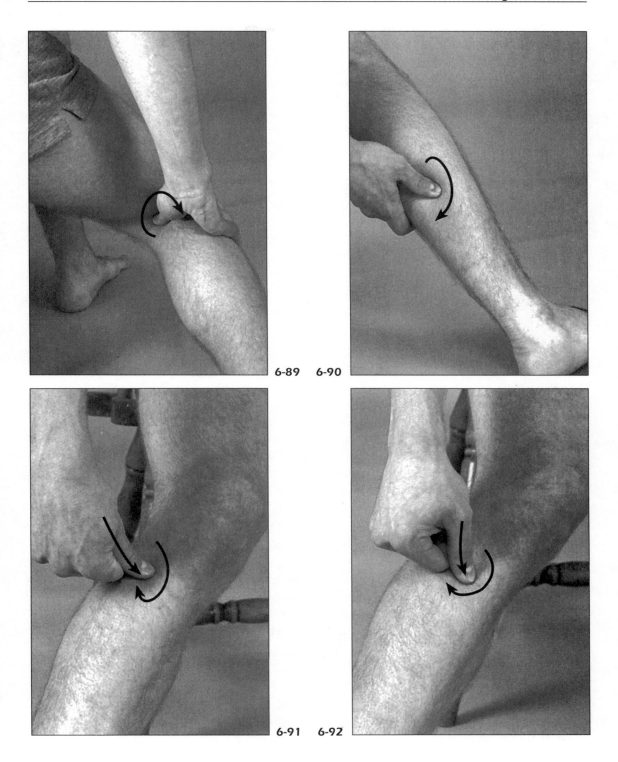

6-89   6-90

6-91   6-92

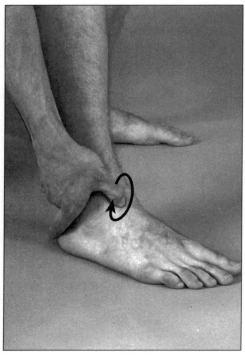
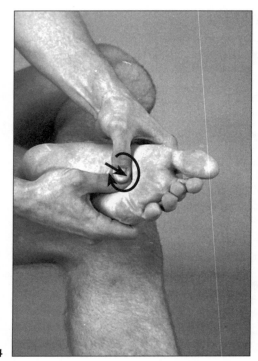

6-93   6-94

Massaging a Patient

When you massage a patient, the basic theory, rules, and techniques are the same as in self massage. The difference is that when you massage a patient, the one being massaged is more relaxed, and you can apply more techniques. Therefore, the treatment can be more effective than self massage.

Step #1. The first step is to loosen up the patient's torso. In order to reach this goal, let the patient lie face down. Next, pull both legs firmly and gently downward (Figure 6-95). This will loosen up the hips and the lower back. Then, pull his arms to loosen the upper back (Figure 6-96). Finally, place your both hands under his pelvis bone and lift the lower back upward (Figure 6-97). This will loosen up the lower back area. In all of these pullings, you may also move from side to side or shake a little bit. The whole idea is to loosen up the back area and make the patient feel comfortable.

Step #2. First grab your patient's shoulder muscles with your thumb and fingers, and rub the muscles forward and backward, vibrating them gently (Figure 6-98). Do not use too much power when you do this, as it will be painful and cause the muscles to tense. This will make the patient more tensed instead of relaxed. After rubbing a few times, the shoulder muscles should be loose and more relaxed. Then press the Jianjing cavity with your thumb or index and middle fingers, and make a circular motion to stimulate the cavity more

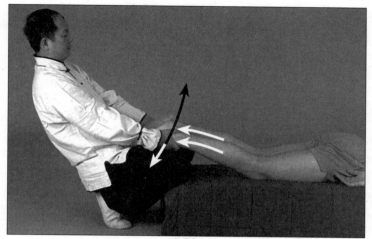

6-95

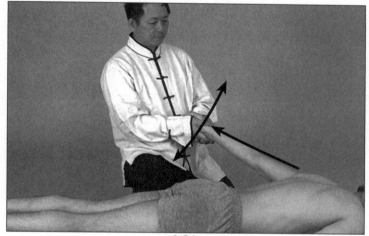

6-96

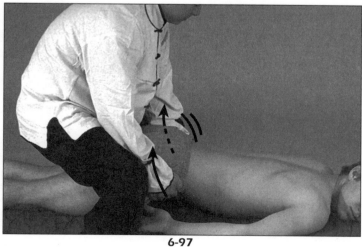

6-97

deeply (Figure 6-99). Finally, circle and slide your hands or the edge of your hands along the shoulder muscles and down to the shoulder joints (Figure 6-100).

Step #3. Use your palm to push from the spine to the sides of the back (Figure 6-101). Start from the upper back and down to the hip area. This will gently stretch and loosen up the center of the back. You may repeat the same process a few times.

Step #4. Use the palm or the edge of the hand to massage the muscles beside the spine (Figures 6-102 and 6-103). This will loosen up the back muscles and make the patient very relaxed.

Step #5. Use your finger tips to gently touch the patient's skin on the back and move down from the upper back to the bottom of the feet and from the upper back to the hands (Figure 6-104). This light touch will help your patient reach a deeper state of relaxation.

Step #6. Use the palms to press downward on the muscles just beside the spine from the upper back to the hips (Figures 6-105 and 6-106). When you are doing so, ask your patient to inhale deeply first and then exhale. While your patient is exhaling, you also exhale and press your palms down at the same time. This will loosen up the ligaments between the joints on the spine.

Step #7. Use your palm or the edge of you palm to rub and massage the lower back area (Figure 6-107). Start with gentle power and after the cells on this area are excited, then apply more power and try to reach deeper.

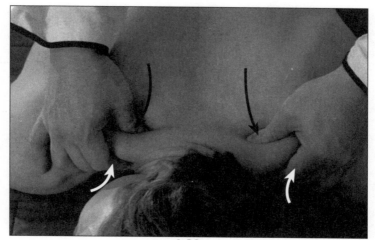

6-98

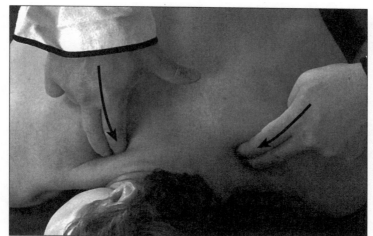

6-99

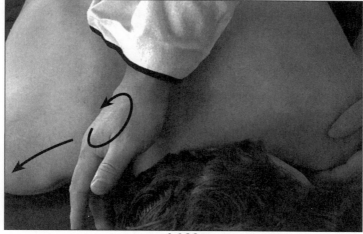

6-100

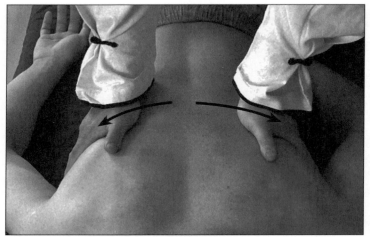

6-101

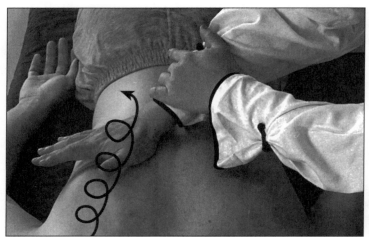

6-102

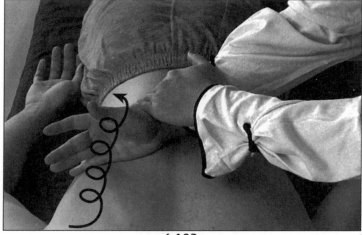

6-103

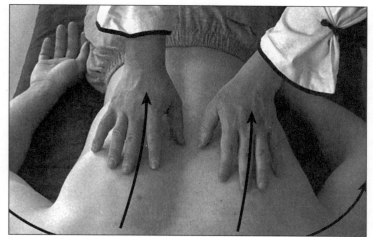

6-104

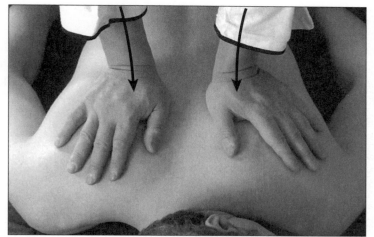

6-105

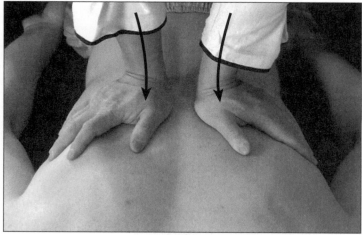

6-106

Step #8. Use the thumb or the base of the palm to gently press and rub the Shenshu (B-23, 腎俞), Mingmen (Gv-4, 命門), Juliao (GB-26, 居髎), Baliao (B-31-34, 八髎)(i.e., sacrum), Changqiang (Gv-1, 長強), Huiyin (Co-1, 會陰), Zhibian (B-49, 秩邊), and Huantiao (GB-30, 環跳) cavities. Repeat for a few times. This process is to improve the Qi and blood circulation by leading the Qi from deep to shallow and from the center to the sides. This effort can help to ease pain in these areas (Figures 6-108 to 6-115).

To massage the sacrum, use the base of your palm or the side of the fist to rub the area with a circular motion. Since this is the junction of the upward Qi and downward Qi, you should circle in both directions the same number of times (Figure 6-112).

When you massage the Changqiang cavity, first use the base of your palm to push inward and upward a few times (Figure 6-113). This will follow the natural Qi circulation which is upward to the back from the Changqiang cavity. This can also lead the Qi to the sacrum and enter the spinal cord and bone marrow in the spine.

When you massage the Huiyin cavity, spread your partner's legs a comfortable distance apart. Press gently on the Huiyin cavity with your middle finger and circle around (Figure 6-115). If your patient feels uncomfortable, you may skip this Huiyin cavity massage.

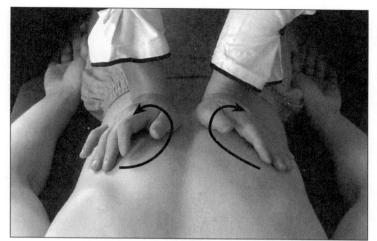

6-107

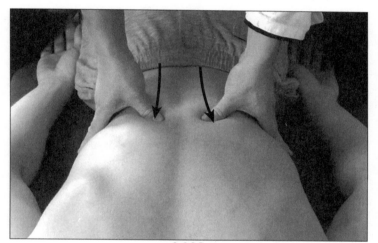

6-108

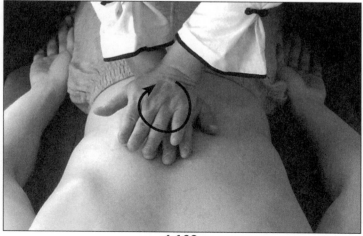

6-109

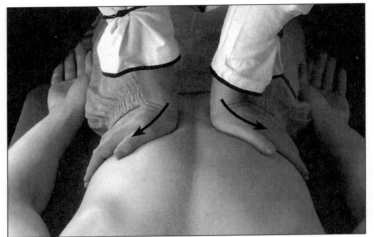

6-110

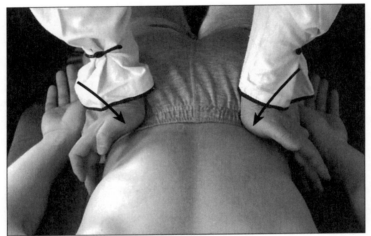

6-111

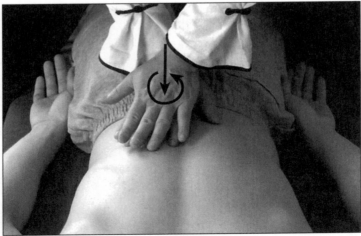

6-112

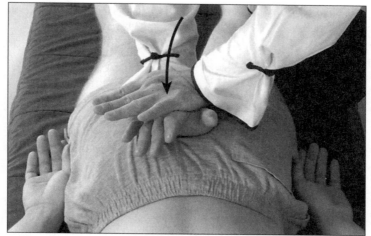

6-113

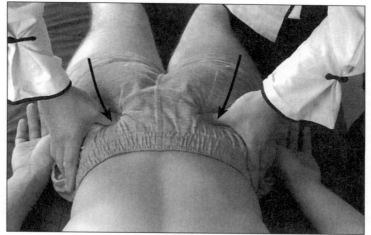

6-114

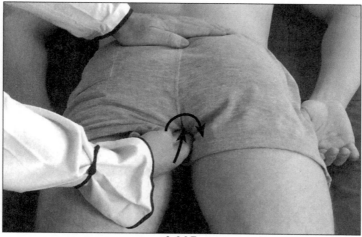

6-115

Step #9. Next, you lead the Qi down to the bottom of the feet. First use the thumb or the edge of the palm to press and rub the Chengfu cavity (B-50, 承扶) for one or two minutes (Figures 6-116 and 6-117). Next, use the thumb to press and rub the Weizhong cavity (B-54, 委中) (Figure 6-118) and the Chengshan cavity (B-57, 承山) for a few minutes (Figure 6-119). Use the thumb or index finger to press and rub the Yanglingquan cavity (GB-34, 陽陵泉) (Figures 6-120 and 6-121) and the Zusanli cavity (S-36, 足三里) (Figures 6-122 and 6-123) for several minutes. Finally, use the thumb to massage the Jiexi cavity (S-41, 解溪) (Figure 6-124), and the Yongquan cavity (K-1, 湧泉) (Figure 6-125) for one or two minutes. Repeat several times. This process is to lead the Qi downward to the bottom of feet.

Step #10. Use the edge of your palms to gently hit your patient from the lower back to the calves a few times (Figure 6-126). Emphasize the hip area and stimulate here longer than other places. This area is the key place to lead the stagnant Qi in the back down to the legs. After hitting stimulation, you should then use your palm to gently rub your patient from the lower back to the calf area (Figure 6-127).

The above massage techniques can ease pain and make your patient more comfortable. After massage, if your patient feels better, you should do the Qigong exercises. Massage can alleviate the pain and make the patient more comfortable, but it does not heal or recondition the problem from the root. Only through strengthening the back, both by adopting the correct life style and consistently performing the Qigong exercises, can the root cause of the pain be eliminated.

References

1. 意在精神，不在氣，在氣則滯。

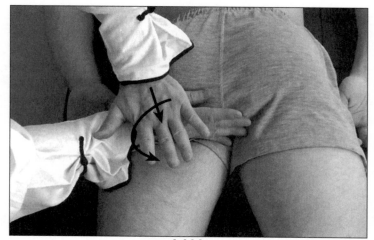

6-116

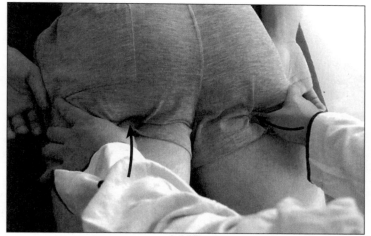

6-117

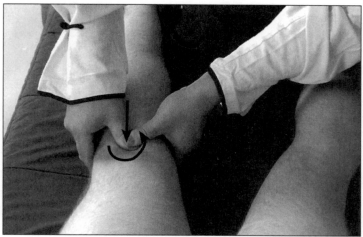

6-118

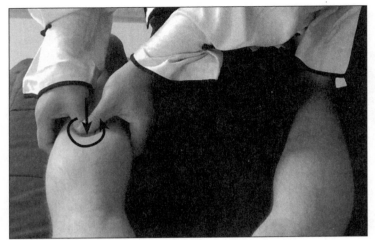

6-119

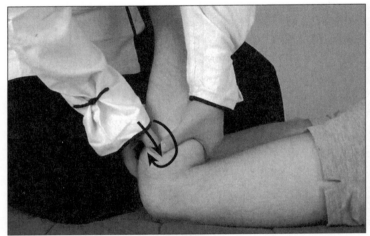

6-120

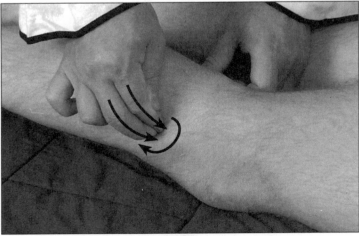

6-121

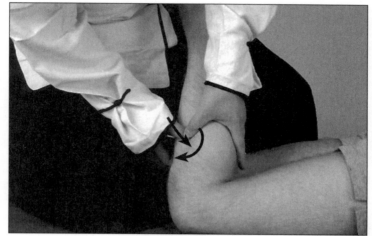

6-122

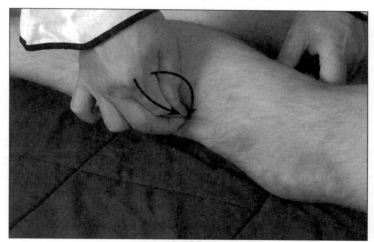

6-123

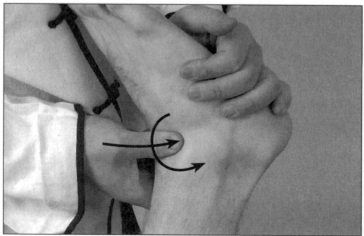

6-124

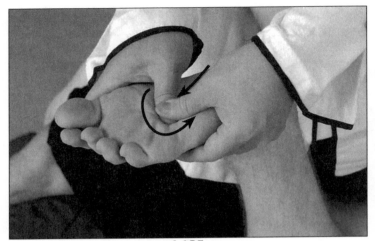

6-125

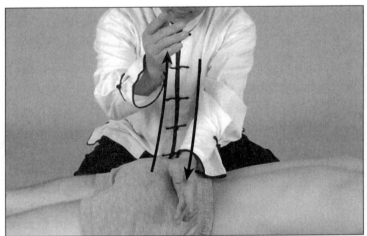

6-126

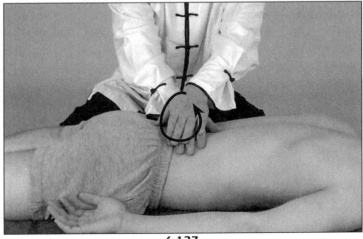

6-127

CHAPTER 7

Conclusion

結論

Again I would like to stress that this book is written based on my personal under-standing and experience both from the Western and Chinese medical point of view about the lower back pain. Moreover, because my personal knowledge and experience in acupuncture and herbal treatments for the same problem is limited, I do not include these two methods of treatment in this book. I sincerely hope quali-fied Chinese physicians will write books about these treatments to remedy this void.

In addition, I would like to urge you to keep your mind open, study, and absorb other sources of information about back pain treatment. The more information you have, the more angles you will have. This will help you analyze the problem more logically and wisely.

Finally, I would like to remind you that the most important part of the entire treat-ment is to rebuild the strength of your torso. This will take a great deal of patience and time. Therefore, the first and the most important challenge you must face is to establish your strong will and confidence. Without these factors, all of the methods you have read in this book will be useless. Proceed with the treatment cautiously and patiently. If you give up you will never make progress. Normally, it will take about three months of Qigong exercise to see primary results. Moreover, in order to main-tain the health of your spine, you should not stop the Qigong exercises even if the symptoms of back pain have gone. Keep yourself in good physical condition and build up a firm and strong spirit. This is the way to prevent and fight disease.

Translation and Glossary of Chinese Terms

Ai 哀 Sorrow.

Ai 愛 Love, kindness.

An Mo 按摩 Literally, "press rub." Together they mean massage.

An Yang, Henan province 河南、安陽 The location of an old Chinese capital during the Shang dynasty (1766-1154 B.C.). It has become an important site for archeological study.

Ba Duan Jin 八段錦 Eight Pieces of Brocade. A Wai Dan Qigong practice which is said to have been created by Marshal Yue Fei during the Southern Song dynasty (1127-1279 A.D.).

Ba Kua (Bagua) 八卦 Literally, "Eight Divinations." Also called the Eight Trigrams. In Chinese philosophy, the eight basic variations. They are shown in the *Yi Jing* as groups of single and broken lines.

Ba Kua Chang (Baguazhang) 八卦掌 Eight Trigrams Palm. One of the internal Qigong martial styles, believed to have been created by Dong, Hai-Chuan between 1866 and 1880 A.D.

Ba Mai 八脈 Referred to as the eight extraordinary vessels. These eight vessels are considered to be Qi reservoirs, which regulate the Qi status in the primary Qi channels.

Bai He 白鶴 Means "White Crane." One of the Chinese southern martial styles.

Baliao (B-31-34) 八髎 Eight cavities on the sacrum which belong to the Bladder Primary Qi Channels. Baliao includes Shangliao, Ciliao, Zhongliao, and Xialiao (four on each side of sacrum).

Bao Pu Zi 抱朴子 A well-known Qigong and Chinese medical book written by Ge Hong during the Jin dynasty in the 3rd century A.D.

Bao Shen Mi Yao 保身祕要 A Qigong and medical book that describes moving and stationary Qigong practices, written by Cao, Yuan-Bai during the Qing dynasty (1644-1911 A.D.).

Bagua (Ba Kua) 八卦 Literally, "Eight Divinations." Also called the Eight Trigrams. In Chinese philosophy, the eight basic variations; shown in the *Yi Jing* as groups of single and broken lines.

Bian Que 扁鵲 A well-known physician who wrote the book *Nan Jing* (*Classic on Disorders*) during the Chinese Qin and Han dynasties (221 B.C.-220 A.D., Ø≥°A∫~).

Bian Shi 砭石 Stone probes that were used to press the acupuncture cavities for healing before metal needles were available.

Cao, Yuan-Bai 曹元白 A well-known physician and Qigong master who wrote a book during the Qing dynasty (1644-1911 A.D.) called *Bao Shen Mi Yao* (*The Secret Important Document of Body Protection*) which describes moving and stationary Qigong practices.

Chan (Ren) 禪，忍 A Chinese school of Mahayana Buddhism which asserts that enlightenment can be attained through meditation, self-contemplation and intuition, rather than through study of scripture. Chan is called Zen in Japan.

Chang 長 Long.

Chang Chuan (Changquan) 長拳 Means "Long Range Fist." Chang Chuan includes all northern Chinese long range martial styles. Chang Chuan has also been used to refer to Taijiquan.

Chang, San-Feng 張三豐 Chang, San-Feng is credited as the creator of Taijiquan during the Song dynasty (960-1127 A.D.) in China.

Chang, Xiang-San 張詳三 A well-known Chinese martial artist in Taiwan.

Changqiang (Gv-1) 長強 Name of an acupuncture cavity that belongs to the Governing Vessel.

Changquan (Chang Chuan) 長拳 Means "Long Range Fist." Changquan includes all northern Chinese long range martial styles. Changquan has also been used to refer to Taijiquan.

Chao, Yuan-Fang 巢元方 A well-known physician and Qigong master during the Sui and Tang dynasties (581-907 A.D.). Chao, Yuan-Fang compiled the *Zhu Bing Yuan Hou Lun* (*Thesis on the Origins and Symptoms of Various Diseases*), which is a veritable encyclopedia of Qigong methods, listing 260 different ways of increasing the Qi flow.

Chen, Ji-Ru 陳繼儒 A well-known physician and Qigong master who wrote the book *Yang Shen Fu Yu* (*Brief Introduction to Nourishing the Body*) about the three treasures: Jing (essence), Qi (internal energy), and Shen (spirit) during Qing dynasty (1644-1911 A.D.).

Chengfu (B-50) 承扶 An acupuncture cavity that belongs to the Bladder Primary Qi Channel.

Cheng, Gin-Gsao 曾金灶 Dr. Yang, Jwing-Ming's White Crane master.

Chi (Qi) 氣 The energy pervading the universe, including the energy circulating in the human body.

Chi Kung (Qigong) 氣功 The Gongfu of Qi, which means the study of Qi.

Chin Na (Qin Na) 擒拿 Literally "grab control." A component of Chinese martial arts which emphasizes grabbing techniques, to control your opponent's joints, in conjunction with attacking certain acupuncture cavities.

Chong Mai 衝脈 Thrusting Vessel. One of the eight extraordinary Qi vessels.

Ciliao (B-32) 次髎 One of four cavities on each side of sacrum belonging to the Bladder Primary Qi Channel.

Confucius 孔子 A Chinese scholar from the period 551-479 B.C., whose philosophy has significantly influenced Chinese culture.

Da Mo 達摩 The Indian Buddhist monk who is credited with creating the Yi Jin Jing and Xi Sui Jing while at the Shaolin monastery. His last name was Sardili and he was also known as Bodhidarma. He was once the prince of a small tribe in southern India.

Da Zhou Tian 大周天 Literally, "Grand Cycle Heaven." Usually translated as Grand Circulation. After a Nei Dan Qigong practitioner completes Small Circulation, he will circulate his Qi through the entire body or exchange the Qi with nature.

Dai Mai 帶脈 Girdle (or Belt) Vessel. One of the eight Qi vessels.

Dan Tian 丹田 Literally, "Field of Elixir." Locations in the body that can store and generate Qi (elixir) in the body. The Upper, Middle, and Lower Dan Tian are located respectively between the eyebrows, at the solar plexus, and a few inches below the navel.

Dan Tian Qi 丹田氣 Usually, the Qi that is converted from Original Essence and is stored in the Lower Dan Tian. This Qi is considered "water Qi" and is able to calm down the body. Also called Xian Tian Qi (Pre-Heaven Qi).

Dao 道 The "way," by implication the "natural way."

Dao De Jing 道德經 Morality Classic. Written by Lao Zi.

Dao Jia 道家 The Dao family. Daoism. Created by Lao Zi during the Zhou dynasty (1122-934 B.C.). In the Han dynasty (c. 58 A.D.), it was mixed with the Buddhism to become the Daoist religion (Dao Jiao).

Dao Jiao 道教 Daoist religion created by Zhang, Dao-Ling who combined the traditional Daoist principles with Buddhism during the Chinese Han dynasty.

Di 地 The Earth. Earth, Heaven (Tian) and Man (Ren) are the "Three Natural Powers" (San Cai).

Di Li Shi 地理師 Di Li means "geomancy" and Shi means "teacher." Therefore Di Li Shi is a teacher or master who analyzes geographic locations according to the formulas in the *Yi Jing* and the energy distributions in the Earth. Also called Feng Shui Shi.

Di Qi 地氣 The Qi or the energy of the planet Earth.

Dian 點 To point or to press.

Dian Mai (Dim Mak) 點脈 Mai means "the blood vessel" (Xue Mai) or "the Qi channel" (Qi Mai). Dian Mai means "To press the blood vessel or Qi channel."

Dian Qi 電氣 Dian means "electricity" and so Dian Qi means "electrical energy" (electricity). In China, a word is often placed before "Qi" to identify the different kinds of energy.

Dian Xue 點穴 Dian means "to point and exert pressure" and Xue means "the cavities." Dian Xue refers to those Qin Na techniques which specialize in attacking acupuncture cavities to immobilize or kill an opponent.

Dian Xue Massages 點穴按摩 A Chinese massage technique in which the acupuncture cavities are stimulated through pressing. Dian Xue massage is also called acupressure and is the root of Japanese Shiatsu.

Dim Mak (Dian Mai) 點脈 Cantonese of "Dian Mai."

Dong, Hai-Chuan 董海川 A well-known Chinese internal martial artist who is credited as the creator of Baguazhang in the late Qing dynasty (1644-1911 A.D.).

Du Mai 督脈 Usually translated "Governing Vessel." One of the eight extraordinary vessels.

Eastern Han Dynasty 東漢 A Chinese dynasty from 25-168 A.D.

Emei 峨嵋 Name of a mountain in Sichuan Province, China.

Er Lu Mai Fu 二路埋伏 Second way to ambush. The name of a Shaolin Long Fist sequence.

Fan Tong Hu Xi 返童呼吸 Back to childhood breathing. Breathing training in Nei Dan Qigong through which the practitioner tries to regain control of the muscles in the lower abdomen. Also called "abdominal breathing."

Feng Shui 風水 Literally, "wind-water."

Feng Shui Shi 風水師 Literally, "wind water teacher." Teacher or master of geomancy. Geomancy is the art or science of analyzing the natural energy relationships in a location, especially the interrelationships between "wind" and "water," hence the name. Also called Di Li Shi.

Ge Hong 葛洪 A famous physician and Qigong master who wrote the book, *Bao Pu Zi* during the Jin dynasty in the 3rd century A.D.

Ge Zhi Yu Lun 格致餘論 Chinese name of the book, *A Further Thesis of Complete Study.* A medical and Qigong thesis written by Zhu, Dan-Xi during the Chinese Song, Jin, and Yuan dynasties (960-1368 A.D.).

Gong (Kung) 功 Energy or hard work.

Gongfu (Kung Fu) 功夫 Means "energy-time." Anything which will take time and energy to learn or to accomplish is called Gongfu.

Gui Qi 鬼氣 The Qi residue of a dead person. It is believed by the Chinese Buddhists and Daoists that this Qi residue is a so-called ghost.

Gung Li Chuan 功力拳 The name of a barehand sequence in Chinese Long Fist martial arts.

Guoshu 國術 Abbreviation of "Zhongguo Wushu," which means "Chinese Martial Techniques."

Han Dynasty 漢朝 A dynasty in Chinese history (206 B.C.-221 A.D.).

Han, Ching-Tang 韓慶堂 A well-known Chinese martial artist, especially in Taiwan in the last forty years. Master Han is also Dr. Yang, Jwing-Ming's Long Fist Grand Master.

He 和 Harmony or peace.

Hen 恨 Hate.

Hou Tian Qi 後天氣 Post-Birth Qi. This Qi is converted from the Essence of food and air and is classified as "fire Qi" since it can make your body too Yang.

Hsing Yi Chuan (Xingyiquan) 形意拳 Literally, "Shape-mind Fist." An internal style of Gongfu in which the mind or thinking determines the shape or movement of the body. Creation of the style is attributed to Marshal Yue Fei.

Hu Bu Gong 虎步功 Tiger Step Gong. A style of Qigong training.

Hua Tuo 華陀 A well-known physician during the Chinese Jin dynasty in the 3rd century A.D.

Huan Jing Bu Nao 還精補腦 Literally, "To return the Essence to nourish the brain." A Daoist Qigong training process wherein Qi that is converted from Essence is led to the brain to nourish it.

Huan 緩 Slow.

Huang Di (2690-2590 B.C.) 黃帝 Yellow Emperor.

Huantiao (GB-30) 環跳 An acupuncture point that belongs to the Gall Bladder Primary Qi Channel.

Huiyin (Co-1) 會陰 An acupuncture cavity belonging to the Conception Vessel.

Huo Long Gong 火龍功 Fire Dragon Gong. A style of Qigong training created by Taiyang martial stylists.

Huo Qi 活氣 Huo means "alive." Huo Qi is the Qi of a living person or animal.

Jia Dan Tian 假丹田 False Dan Tian. Daoists believe that the Lower Dan Tian located on the front side of abdomen is not the real Dan Tian. The real Dan Tian corresponds to the physical center of gravity. The False Dan Tian is called Qihai (Qi ocean) in Chinese medicine.

Jia Gu Wen 甲骨文 Oracle-Bone Scripture. Earliest evidence of the Chinese use of the written word. Found on pieces of turtle shell and animal bone from the Shang dynasty (1766-1154 B.C.). Most of the information recorded was of a religious nature.

Jianjing (GB-21) 肩井 An acupuncture cavity belonging to the Gall Bladder Primary Qi Channel.

Jiao Hua Gong 叫化功 Beggar Gong. A style of Qigong training.

Jiexi (S-41) 解溪 An acupuncture cavity belonging to the Stomach Primary Qi Channel.

Jin 筋 Means "tendons."

Jin Dynasty 晉 A Chinese dynasty in the 3rd century A.D.

Jin Kui Yao Lue 金匱要略 A Chinese book named *Prescriptions from the Golden Chamber*, which discusses the use of breathing and acupuncture to maintain good Qi flow. This book was written by Zhang, Zhong-Jing during the Chinese Qin and Han dynasties (221 B.C.-220 A.D.).

Jin Zhong Zhao 金鐘罩 Literally, "golden bell cover." A higher level of Iron Shirt training.

Jin, Shao-Feng 金紹峰 Dr. Yang, Jwing-Ming's White Crane grand master.

Jing 精 Essence. The most refined part of anything.

Jing 靜 Calm and silent.

Jing 經 Channels. Sometimes translated as "meridians." Jing refers to the twelve organ-related "rivers" that circulate Qi throughout the body.

Jing Zi 精子 Literally, "essence son." The most refined part of human essence. The sperm.

Juliao (GB-29) 居髎 An acupuncture cavity belonging to the Gall Bladder Primary Qi Channel.

Jun Qing 君倩 A Daoist and Chinese doctor from the Chinese Jin dynasty (265-420 A.D.). Jun Qing is credited as the creator of the Five Animal Sports Qigong practice.

Kan 坎 One of the Eight Trigrams.

Kao Tao 高濤 Master Yang, Jwing-Ming's first Taijiquan master.

Karate 空手道 Literally, "barehand." Karate Do is "the barehand way." A Japanese martial art rooted in Chinese Southern White Crane.

Kong Qi 空氣 Air.

Kun 坤 One of the Eight Trigrams.

Kung (Gong) 功 Means "energy" or "hard work."

Kung Fu (Gongfu) 功夫 Literally, "energy-time." Any study, learning, or practice that requires a lot of patience, energy, and time to complete. Since practicing Chinese martial arts requires a great deal of time and energy, Chinese martial arts are commonly called Gongfu.

Kuoshu (Guoshu) 國術 Literally, "national techniques." Another name for Chinese martial arts. First used by President Chiang, Kai-Shek in 1926 at the founding of the Nanking Central Guoshu Institute.

La Ma 喇嘛 A Tibetan monk. Also used for Tibetan White Crane style.

Lan Shi Mi Cang 蘭室祕藏 *Secret Library of the Orchid Room*. Name of a Chinese medical and Qigong book written by Li Guo during the Song, Jin, and Yuan dynasties (960-1368 A.D.).

Lao Zi 老子 The creator of Daoism, also called Li Er.

Laogong (P-8) 勞宮 Cavity name. The Laogong is on the Pericardium Channel in the center of the palm.

Le 樂 Joy or happiness.

Li 離 A phase of the Bagua (Eight Trigrams), Li represents fire.

Li Er 李耳 Nick-name of Lao Zi, the creator of scholarly Daoism.

Li Guo 李果 A well-known Chinese physician and Qigong master who wrote the book, *Lan Shi Mi Cang (Secret Library of the Orchid Room)* during the Song, Jin, and Yuan dynasties (960-1368 A.D.).

Li, Mao-Ching 李茂清 Dr. Yang, Jwing-Ming's Long Fist master.

Lian Jing Hua Qi 練精化氣 To refine the Essence and convert it into Qi. One of the Qigong training processes through which you convert Essence into Qi.

Lian Qi 練氣 Lian means "To train, to strengthen and to refine." A Daoist training process through which your Qi grows stronger and more abundant.

Lian Qi Hua Shen 練氣化神 To refine the Qi to nourish the spirit. Part of the Qigong training process in which you learn how to lead Qi to the head to nourish the brain and Shen (spirit).

Lian Shen 練神 To train the spirit. To refine and strengthen the Shen and make it more focused.

Lian Shen Fan Xu 練神返虛 To refine the Shen into emptiness. Part of the Daoist Qigong training process in which you learn how to lead your Shen (spirit) into the emptiness (i.e. freedom from emotional bondage.)

Lian Shen Liao Xing 練神了性 To refine the spirit and end human nature. This is the final stage of spiritual Qigong training for enlightenment. In this process you learn to keep your emotions neutral and try to be undisturbed by human nature.

Liang Dynasty 梁 A dynasty in Chinese history (502-557 A.D.)

Lien Bu Chuan 連步拳 One of the basic Long Fist barehand sequences.

Ling Shu 靈樞 A well-known Chinese physician who wrote a medical book called *Huang Di Nei Jing Su Wen* (*The Yellow Emperor's Classic*) during the Han dynasty (circa 100-300 B.C.).

Lingtai (Gv-10) 靈台 An acupuncture cavity belonging to the Governing Vessel.

Liu He Ba Fa 六合八法 Literally, "Six combinations eight methods." One of the Chinese internal martial arts, its techniques are combined from Taijiquan, Xingyi and Baguazhang. This internal martial art was reportedly created by Chen Bo during the Song dynasty (960-1279 A.D.).

Luo 絡 The small Qi channels which branch out from the primary Qi channels and are connected to the skin and to the bone marrow.

Mai 脈 Means "vessel" or "Qi channel."

Mencius (372-289 B.C.) 孟子 A well-known scholar who followed the philosophy of Confucius during the Chinese Zhou dynasty (909-255 B.C.).

Mian 綿 Soft.

Ming dynasty 明朝 A Chinese dynasty from 1368 to 1644 A.D.

Mingmen (Gv-4) 命門 Name of an acupuncture cavity belonging to the Governing Vessel.

Na 拿 Means "to hold" or "to grab."

Nan Hua Jing 南華經 A book written by the Daoist philosopher Zhuang Zi around 300 B.C. This book describes the relationship between health and the breath.

Nan Jing 難經 *Classic on Disorders*. A medical book written by the famous physician Bian Que during the Qin and Han dynasties (221 B.C.-220 A.D.). *Nan Jing* describes methods of using the breathing to increase Qi circulation.

Nei Dan 內丹 Literally, "Internal elixir." A form of Qigong in which Qi (the elixir) is built up in the body and spread out to the limbs.

Nei Gong Tu Shuo 内功圖説 *Illustrated Explanation of Nei Gong.* A Qigong book written by Wang, Zu-Yuan during the Qing dynasty. This book presents the Twelve Pieces of Brocade and explains the idea of combining both moving and stationary Qigong.

Nei Jing 内經 *Inner Classic.* A Chinese medical book written during the reign of the Yellow emperor (2690-2590 B.C.).

Nei Shi Fan Ting 内視返聽 Means "To see internally and to listen inwardly."

Nei Shi Gongfu 内視功夫 Nei Shi means "To look internally," so Nei Shi Gongfu refers to the art of looking inside yourself to read the state of your health and the condition of your Qi.

Nei Wai He Yi 内外合一 Literally, "Internal and external unified as one." Means the unification of the external action and the internal Qi.

Nei Wai Xie He 内外諧合 Literally, "Internal and external harmonized." Means the harmonious coordination of physical action and the internal mind and Qi.

Nu 怒 Anger.

Ping 平 Peace and harmony.

Pu Tong An Mo 普通按摩 General massage. The massage for physical and mental relaxation and enjoyment.

Qi (Chi) 氣 The general definition of Qi is: universal energy, including heat, light, and electromagnetic energy. A narrower definition of Qi refers to the energy circulating in human or animal bodies. A current popular model is that the Qi circulating in the human body is bioelectric in nature.

Qi An Mo 氣按摩 Qi massage. One of the highest levels of massage techniques in which a massage doctor will use his or her Qi to remove the Qi stagnation in a patient's body. Qi massage is also called "Wai Qi Liao Fa" which means "Healing with the external Qi."

Qi Hua Lun 氣化論 Qi variation thesis. An ancient treatise which discusses the variations of Qi in the universe.

Qi Huo 起火 To start the fire. In Qigong practice, it refers to building up Qi at the Lower Dan Tian.

Qi Jing Ba Mai 奇經八脈 Literally, "Strange (odd) channels eight vessels." Usually referred to as the eight extraordinary vessels or simply as the vessels. Called odd or strange because they are not well understood and some of them do not exist in pairs.

Qi Jing Ba Mai Kao 奇經八脈考 *Deep Study of the Extraordinary Eight Vessels.* A book written by Li, Shi-Zhen.

Qi Qing Liu Yu 七情六慾 Seven emotions and six desires. The seven emotions are happiness, anger, sorrow, joy, love, hate and desire. The six desires are the six sensory pleasures associated with the eyes, nose, ears, tongue, body and mind.

Qi Shi 氣勢   Shi means the way something looks or feels. Therefore, the feeling of Qi as it expresses itself.

Qi-Xue 氣血   Literally, "Qi blood." According to Chinese medicine, Qi and blood cannot be separated in our body and so the two words are commonly used together.

Qie Zhen 切診   Palpation. One of the diagnostic techniques used in Chinese medicine.

Qigong (Chi Kung) 氣功   Gong means Gongfu (literally "energy-time"). Therefore, Qigong means study, research, and/or practices related to Qi.

Qigong An Mo 氣功按摩   Qigong massage.

Qihai (Co-6) 氣海   An acupuncture cavity belonging to the Conception Vessel.

Qin Dynasty 秦朝   A Chinese dynasty from 255-206 B.C.

Qin Na (Chin Na) 擒拿   Literally means "grab control." A component of Chinese martial arts which emphasizes grabbing techniques to control your opponent's joints, in conjunction with attacking certain acupuncture cavities.

Qing Dynasty 清朝   A dynasty in Chinese history. The last Chinese dynasty (1644-1912 A.D.).

Re Qi 熱氣   Re means "warmth" or "heat." Generally, Re Qi is used to represent heat. It is used sometimes to imply that a person or animal is still alive since the body is warm.

Rou 揉   Rub. A common massage technique.

Ren 人   Man or mankind.

Ren 仁   Humanity, kindness or benevolence.

Ren Mai 任脈   Conception Vessel. One of the Eight Extraordinary Vessels.

Ren Qi 人氣   Human Qi.

Ren Shi 人事   Literally, "Human relations." Human events, activities and relationships.

Ren Zong 仁宗   One of the Song emperors during the period 1023-1064 A.D.

Ru Jia 儒家   Literally, "Confucian family." Scholars following Confucian thoughts; Confucianists.

Ru Men Shi Shi 儒門視事   *The Confucian Point of View.* A book written by Zhang, Zi-He during the Song, Jin, and Yuan dynasties (960-1368 A.D.).

San Bao 三寶   Three treasures. Essence (Jing), energy (Qi) and spirit (Shen). Also called San Yuan (three origins).

San Ben 三本   The Three Foundations.

San Cai 三才   Three powers. The three powers are Heaven, Earth and Man.

San Gong 散功 Literally, "Energy dispersion." A state of premature degeneration of the muscles where the Qi cannot effectively energize them. It can be caused by earlier over-training.

San Yuan 三元 Three origins. Also called "San Bao" (three treasures). Human Essence (Jing), energy (Qi) and spirit (Shen).

Shang Dan Tian 上丹田 Upper Dan Tian. Located at the third eye, it is the residence of the Shen (spirit).

Shang dynasty 商朝 A dynasty in Chinese history from 1766-1154 B.C.

Shangliao (B-31) 上髎 One of four cavities on each side of the sacrum belonging to the Bladder Primary Qi Channel.

Shaolin 少林 Young woods. Name of the Shaolin Temple.

Shaolin Temple 少林寺 A monastery located in Henan Province, China. The Shaolin Temple is well known because of its martial arts training.

Shen 神 Spirit. According to Chinese Qigong, the Shen resides at the Upper Dan Tian (the third eye).

Shen 深 Deep.

Shen Tai 神胎 Spiritual embryo. It is also called "Ling Tai."

Shen Xin Ping Heng 身心平衡 Body and heart (mind) balanced. This means a balance between the physical body and the mental body.

Sheng Tai 聖胎 Holy embryo. Another name for the spiritual embryo (Shen Tai).

Shenshu (B-23) 腎俞 Name of an acupuncture cavity belonging to the Bladder Qi Channel.

Shi Er Jing 十二經 The Twelve Primary Qi Channels in Chinese medicine.

Shi Er Zhuang 十二庄 Twelve Postures. A style of Qigong practice created during the Chinese Qing dynasty.

Shi Ji 史紀 Historical Record. A book written in the Spring and Autumn and Warring States Periods (770-221 B.C.).

Shou Jue Yin Xin Bao Luo Jing 手厥陰心包絡經 Arm Absolute Yin Pericardium Channel. One of the twelve primary Qi channels.

Shou Shao Yang San Jiao Jing 手少陽三焦經 Arm Lesser Yang Triple Burner Channel. One of the twelve primary Qi channels.

Shou Shao Yin Xin Jing 手少陰心經 Arm Lesser Yin Heart Channel. One of the twelve primary Qi channels.

Shou Tai Yang Xiao Chang Jing 手太陽小腸經 Arm Greater Yang Small Intestine Channel. One of the twelve primary Qi channels.

Shou Tai Yin Fei Jing 手太陰肺經 Arm Greater Yin Lung Channel. One of the twelve primary Qi channels.

Shou Yang Ming Da Chang Jing 手陽明大腸經 Arm Yang Brightness Large Intestine Channel. One of the twelve primary Qi channels.

Si Qi 死氣 Dead Qi. The Qi remaining in a dead body. Sometimes called "ghost Qi" (Gui Qi).

Song Dynasty 宋朝 A dynasty in Chinese history (960-1279 A.D.).

Southern Song Dynasty 南宋 After the Song dynasty was conquered by the Jin race from Mongolia, the Song people moved to the south and established another country, called Southern Song (1127-1279 A.D.).

Su Wen 素問 The name of a medical book. The complete name of the book is called *Huang Di Nei Jing Su Wen* (*The Yellow Emperor's Classic*). This book was written by Ling Shu during the Chinese Han dynasty (circa 100-300 B.C.).

Suan Ming Shi 算命師 Literally, "Calculate life teacher." A fortune teller who is able to calculate your future and destiny.

Sui Dynasty 隋 A dynasty in China during the period of 581-618 A.D.

Sun, Si-Ma 孫思邈 A well-known Chinese physician and Qigong master who wrote the book *Qian Jin Fang* (*Thousand Gold Prescriptions*) during the Sui and Tang dynasties (581-907 A.D.).

Tai Chi Chuan (Taijiquan) 太極拳 A Chinese internal martial style based on the theory of Taiji (Grand ultimate).

Taiji 太極 Means "Grand ultimate." It is this force which generates two poles, Yin and Yang.

Taijiquan (Tai Chi Chuan) 太極拳 A Chinese internal martial style based on the theory of Taiji (Grand ultimate).

Taipei 台北 The capital city of Taiwan located in the north.

Taiwan 台灣 An island to the south-east of mainland China. Also known as Formosa.

Taiwan University 台灣大學 A well-known university located in northern Taiwan.

Taiyang Martial Stylists 太陽宗 A school of Chinese martial arts that practices Huo Long Gong (Fire Dragon Gong) Qigong training.

Taizuquan 太祖拳 A style of Chinese external martial arts.

Tang Dynasty 唐朝 A dynasty in Chinese history from 618-907 A.D.

Tamkang 淡江 Name of a university in Taiwan.

Tamkang College Guoshu Club 淡江國術社 A Chinese martial arts club founded by Dr. Yang when he was studying in Tamkang College.

Tao, Hong-Jing 陶弘景 A well-known physician and Qigong master who compiled the book *Yang Shen Yan Ming Lu* (*Records of Nourishing the Body and Extending Life*) during 420 to 581 A.D.

Tian 天 Heaven or sky. In ancient China, people believed that Heaven was the most powerful natural energy in this universe.

Tian Qi 天氣 Heaven Qi. It is now commonly used to mean the weather, since weather is governed by Heaven Qi.

Tian Ren He Yi 天人合一 Literally, "Heaven and man unified as one." A high level of Qigong practice in which a Qigong practitioner, through meditation, is able to communicate his Qi with heaven's Qi.

Tian Shi 天時 Heavenly timing. The repeated natural cycles generated by the heavens such as: seasons, months, days and hours.

Tiao Qi 調氣 To regulate the Qi.

Tiao Shen 調身 To regulate the body.

Tiao Shen 調神 To regulate the spirit.

Tiao Xi 調息 To regulate the breathing.

Tiao Xin 調心 To regulate the emotional mind.

Tie Ban Qiao 鐵板橋 Literally, "Iron Board Bridge." Special martial arts strength and endurance training for the torso.

Tie Bu Shan 鐵布衫 Iron shirt. Gongfu training which toughens the body externally and internally.

Tie Sha Zhang 鐵砂掌 Literally, "Iron Sand Palm." A special martial arts conditioning for the palms.

Tong Ren Yu Xue Zhen Jiu Tu 銅人俞穴鍼灸圖 *Illustration of the Brass Man Acupuncture and Moxibustion*. Name of an acupuncture book written by Dr. Wang, Wei-Yi during the Song dynasty.

Tui 推 Push. A major technique in Chinese Tui Na Qigong massage.

Tui Na 推拿 Means "To push and grab." A category of Chinese massages for healing and injury treatment.

Wai Dan 外丹 External elixir. External Qigong exercises in which a practitioner will build up the Qi in his limbs and then lead it into the center of the body for nourishment.

Wai Dan Chi Kung (Wai Dan Qigong) 外丹氣功 External Elixir Qigong. In Wai Dan Qigong, a practitioner will generate Qi to the limbs and then allow the Qi to flow inward to nourish the internal organs.

Wai Jia 外家 External family. Those martial schools which practice the external styles of Chinese martial arts.

Wai Qi Liao Fa 外氣療法 Literally, "External Qi healing." One of the high levels of Qi massage in which a doctor will use his or her Qi to remove Qi stagnation in the patient.

Wai Tai Mi Yao 外台祕要 *The Extra Important Secret*. A Chinese medical book written by Wang Tao during the Sui and Tang dynasties (581-907 A.D.). This book discusses the use of breathing and herbal therapies for disorders of Qi circulation.

Wang Tao 王燾 A well-known Chinese physician and Qigong master who wrote the book, *Wai Tai Mi Yao* (*The Extra Important Secret*) during the Sui and Tang dynasties (581-907 A.D.).

Wang Zhen 望診 Looking. One of the diagnostic techniques used in Chinese medicine.

Wang, Fan-An 汪汎庵 A well-known Chinese physician who wrote the book, *Yi Fan Ji Jie* (*The Total Introduction to Medical Prescriptions*) during the Qing dynasty.

Wang, Wei-Yi 王唯一 A well-known Chinese physician who wrote the book, *Tong Ren Yu Xue Zhen Jiu Tu* (*Illustration of the Brass Man Acupuncture and Moxibustion*) during the Song dynasty.

Wang, Zu-Yuan 王祖源 A well-known Chinese physician who wrote the book, *Nei Gong Tu Shuo* (*Illustrated Explanation of Nei Gong*) during the Qing dynasty.

Wei Qi 衛氣 Protective Qi or Guardian Qi. The Qi at the surface of the body which generates a shield to protect the body from negative external influences such as colds.

Wei, Bo-Yang 魏伯陽 A well-known physician who wrote the book, *Zhou Yi Can Tong Qi* (*A Comparative Study of the Zhou (dynasty) Book of Changes*) during the Qin and Han dynasties (221 B.C.-220 A.D.).

Weizhong (B-54) 委中 An acupuncture cavity belonging to the Bladder Primary Qi Channel.

Wen Zhen 問診 Asking. One of the diagnostic techniques used in Chinese medicine.

Wen Zhen 聞診 Listening and Smelling. Two of the diagnostic techniques used in Chinese medicine.

Wilson Chen 陳威伸 Dr. Yang, Jwing-Ming's friend.

Wu Qin Shi 五禽戲 Five Animal Sports. A set of medical Qigong practices created by Jun Qing during Chinese Jin dynasty (265-420 A.D.).

Wu Tiao 五調 Five regulating methods in Qigong practice which include: regulating the body, regulating the breathing, regulating the mind, regulating the Qi, and regulating the spirit.

Wudang Mountain 武當山 Located in Fubei Province in China.

Wuji 無極 Means "No extremity."

Wuji Qigong 無極氣功 A style of Taiji Qigong practice.

Wushu 武術 Literally, "Martial techniques." A common name for the Chinese martial arts. Many other terms are used, including: Wuyi (martial arts), Wugong (martial Gongfu), Guoshu (national techniques), and Gongfu (energy-time). Because Wushu has been modified in mainland China over the past forty years into gymnastic martial performance, many traditional Chinese martial artist have given up this name in order to avoid confusing modern Wushu with traditional Wushu. Recently, mainland China has attempted to bring modern Wushu back toward its traditional training and practice.

Xi 細 Slender.

Xi 喜 Joy, delight and happiness.

Xi Sui Gong 洗髓功 Gongfu for marrow and brain washing Qigong practice.

Xi Sui Jing 洗髓經 **Literally,** *"Washing Marrow/Brain Classic,"* usually translated *Marrow/Brain Washing Classic*. A Qigong training which specializes in leading Qi to the marrow to cleanse it, or to the brain to nourish the spirit for enlightenment. It is believed that Xi Sui Jing training is the key to longevity and achieving spiritual enlightenment.

Xia Dan Tian 下丹田 Lower Dan Tian. Located in the lower abdomen, it is believed to be the residence of water Qi (Original Qi).

Xialiao (B-34) 下髎 One of four cavities on each side of the sacrum belonging to the Bladder Primary Qi Channel.

Xian Gu 仙骨 Means "Immortal bone." The sacrum is called immortal bone in Daoist Qigong practice.

Xian Tian Qi 先天氣 Pre-Birth Qi or Pre-Heaven Qi. Also called Dan Tian Qi. The Qi that is converted from Original Essence and is stored in the Lower Dan Tian. Considered to be "water Qi," it is able to calm the body.

Xiao 孝 Filial Piety.

Xiao Zhou Tian 小周天 Literally, "Small heavenly cycle." Also called Small Circulation. In Qigong, when you can use your mind to lead Qi through the Conception and Governing Vessels, you have completed Xiao Zhou Tian.

Xin 心 Means "Heart." Xin means the mind generated from emotional disturbance.

Xin 信 Trust.

Xin Xi Xiang Yi 心息相依 Heart (mind) and breathing (are) mutually dependent.

Xingyiquan (Hsing Yi Chuan) 形意拳 Literally, "Shape-mind Fist." An internal style of Gongfu in which the mind or thinking determines the shape or movement of the body. Creation of the style is attributed to Marshal Yue Fei.

Xinzhu Xian 新竹縣 Birthplace of Dr. Yang, Jwing-Ming in Taiwan.

Xiu Qi 修氣 Cultivate the Qi. Cultivate implies to protect, maintain and refine. A Buddhist Qigong training.

Yan 言 Talking or speaking.

Yang 陽 In Chinese philosophy, the active, positive, masculine polarity. In Chinese medicine, Yang means excessive, overactive, overheated. The Yang (or outer) organs are the Gall Bladder, Small Intestine, Large Intestine, Stomach, Bladder, and Triple Burner.

Yang Shen Fu Yu 養生膚語 *Brief Introduction to Nourishing the Body.* A book written by Chen, Ji-Ru during the Qing dynasty.

Yang Shen Jue 養生訣 *Life Nourishing Secrets.* A medical book written by Zhang, An-Dao during the Song, Jin, and Yuan dynasties (960-1368 A.D.).

Yang Shen Yan Ming Lu 養身延命錄 *Records of Nourishing the Body and Extending Life.* A Chinese medical book written by Dao, Hong-Jing in the period 420 to 581 A.D.

Yang, Jwing-Ming 楊俊敏 Author of this book.

Yangchiao Mai 陽蹺脈 Yang Heel Vessel. One of the eight Qi vessels.

Yanglingquan (GB-34) 陽陵泉 An acupuncture cavity belonging to the Gall Bladder Primary Qi Channel.

Yangwei Mai 陽維脈 Yang Linking Vessel. One of the eight vessels.

Yaobeitengtong 腰背疼痛 Means pain in the back and loin; lumbago and back pain. Chinese medical terminology.

Yaojitong 腰脊痛 Means pain along the spinal column. Chinese medical terminology.

Yaokaotong 腰尻痛 Means lumbosacral pain. Chinese medical terminology.

Yaosuan 腰酸 Means soreness of waist. Chinese medical termonology.

Yaotong 腰痛 Means lumbago. Chinese medical termonology.

Yi 意 Mind. Specifically, the mind that is generated by clear thinking and judgment, and which is able to make you calm, peaceful, and wise.

Yi 義 Justice or righteousness.

Yi Fan Ji Jie 醫方集介 *The Total Introduction to Medical Prescriptions.* A Chinese medical book written by Wang, Fan-An during the Qing dynasty.

Yi Jin Jing 易筋經 Literally, "Changing Muscle/Tendon Classic," usually called *The Muscle/Tendon Changing Classic.* Credited to Da Mo around 550 A.D., this work discusses Wai Dan Qigong training for strengthening the physical body.

Yi Jing 易經 *Book of Changes*. A book of divination written during the Zhou dynasty (1122-255 B.C.).

Yi Lu Mai Fa 一路埋伏 A Long Fist middle level sequence.

Yi Shen Yu Qi 以神馭氣 Use the Shen (spirit) to govern the Qi. A Qigong technique. Since the Shen is the headquarters for the Qi, it is the most effective way to control it.

Yi Shou Dan Tian 意守丹田 Keep your Yi on your Lower Dan Tian. In Qigong training, you keep your mind at the Lower Dan Tian in order to build up Qi. When you are circulating your Qi, you always lead your Qi back to your Lower Dan Tian before you stop.

Yi Yi Yin Qi 以意引氣 Use your Yi (wisdom mind) to lead your Qi. A Qigong technique. Yi cannot be pushed, but it can be led. This is best done with the Yi.

Yin 陰 In Chinese philosophy, the passive, negative, feminine polarity. In Chinese medicine, Yin means deficient. The Yin (internal) organs are the Heart, Lungs, Liver, Kidneys, Spleen, and Pericardium.

Yin Xu 殷墟 An archeological dig site of a late Shang dynasty burial ground.

Yinchiao Mai 陰蹻脈 The Yin Heel Vessel. One of the eight vessels.

Ying Gong 硬功 Hard Gongfu. Any Chinese martial training which emphasizes physical strength and power.

Yinwei Mai 陰維脈 Yin Linking Vessel. One of the eight vessels.

Yongquan (K-1) 湧泉 Bubbling Well. Name of an acupuncture cavity belonging to the Kidney Primary Qi Channel.

You 悠 Long, far, meditative, continuous, slow and soft.

Yu 慾 Desire.

Yuan dynasty 元代 A Chinese dynasty from 1206-1367 A.D.

Yuan Jing 元精 Original Essence. The fundamental, original substance inherited from your parents, it is converted into Original Qi.

Yuan Qi 元氣 Original Qi. The Qi created from the Original Essence inherited from your parents.

Yue Fei 岳飛 A Chinese hero in the Southern Song dynasty (1127-1279 A.D.). He is said to have created Ba Duan Jin, Xingyiquan and Yue's Ying Zhua.

Yun 勻 Uniform or even.

Zen (Chan) 忍(禪) Means " To endure." The Japanese name of Chan.

Zhang, An-Dao 張安道 A well-known Chinese physician and Qigong master who wrote the book, *Yang Shen Jue* (*Life Nourishing Secrets*), during the Song, Jin, and Yuan dynasties (960-1368 A.D.).

Zhang, Dao-Ling 張道陵 A Daoist who combined scholarly Daoism with Buddhist philosophies and created Religious Daoism (Dao Jiao) during the Chinese Eastern Han dynasty (25-221 A.D.).

Zhang, Zhong-Jing 張仲景 A well-known Chinese physician who wrote the book, *Jin Kui Yao Lue* (*Prescriptions from the Golden Chamber*), during the Qin and Han dynasties (221 B.C.-220 A.D.).

Zhang, Zi-He 張子和 A well-known Chinese physician who wrote the book, *Ru Men Shi Shi* (*The Confucian Point of View*), during the Song, Jin, and Yuan dynasties (960-1368 A.D.).

Zhen Dan Tian 眞丹田 The Real Dan Tian, which is located at the physical center of gravity.

Zheng Fu Hu Xi 正腹呼吸 Formal Abdominal Breathing. More commonly called Buddhist Breathing.

Zheng Hu Xi 正呼吸 Formal Breathing. More commonly called Buddhist Breathing.

Zheng Qi 正氣 Righteous Qi. When a person is righteous, it is said that he has righteous Qi which evil Qi cannot overcome.

Zhibian (B-49) 秩邊 An acupuncture cavity belonging to the Bladder Primary Qi Channel.

Zhong 忠 Loyalty.

Zhong Dan Tian 中丹田 Middle Dan Tian. Located in the area of the solar plexus, it is the residence of fire Qi.

Zhongliao (B-33) 中髎 One of four cavities on each side of the sacrum belonging to the Bladder Primary Qi Channel.

Zhou dynasty 周朝 A dynasty in China during period of 1122-934 B.C.

Zhou Yi Can Tong Qi 周易參同契 *A Comparative Study of the Zhou (dynasty) Book of Changes*. A medical and Qigong book written by Wei, Bo-Yang during the Qin and Han dynasties (221 B.C.-220 A.D.).

Zhu Bing Yuan Hou Lun 諸病源候論 *Thesis on the Origins and Symptoms of Various Diseases*. A Chinese medical book written by Chao, Yuan-Fang during the Sui and Tang dynasties (581-907 A.D.).

Zhu, Dan-Xi 朱丹溪 A well-known Chinese physician who wrote the book, *Ge Zhi Yu Lun* (*A Further Thesis of Complete Study*), during the Song, Jin, and Yuan dynasties (960-1368 A.D.).

Zhuan Qi Zhi Rou 專氣致柔 Means "Concentrate on Qi and achieve softness." A famous sentence written in Lao Zi's *Dao De Jing*.

Zhuang Zhou 莊周 A contemporary of Mencius who advocated Daoism.

Zhuang Zi 莊子 Zhuang Zhou. A contemporary of Mencius who advocated Daoism. Zhuang Zi also means the works of Zhuang Zhou.

Zu Jue Yin Gan Jing 足厥陰肝經 Leg Absolute Yin Liver Channel. One of the twelve primary Qi channels.

Zu Shao Yang Dan Jing 足少陽膽經 Leg Lesser Yang Gall Bladder Channel. One of the twelve primary Qi channels.

Zu Shao Yin Shen Jing 足少陰腎經 Leg Lesser Yin Kidney Channel. One of the twelve primary Qi channels.

Zu Tai Yang Pang Guang Jing 足太陽膀胱經 Leg Greater Yang Bladder Channel. One of the twelve primary Qi channels.

Zu Tai Yin Pi Jing 足太陰脾經 Leg Greater Yin Spleen Channel. One of the twelve primary Qi channels.

Zu Yang Ming Wei Jing 足陽明胃經 Leg Yang Brightness Stomach Channel. One of the twelve primary Qi channels.

Zusanli (S-36) 足三里 An acupuncture cavity belonging to the Stomach Primary Qi Channel.

INDEX

Books & Videos from YMAA

YMAA Publication Center Books

YMAA Publication Center Children's Books

YMAA Publication Center Videotapes

YMAA Publication Center 楊氏武藝協會

38 Hyde Park Avenue • Jamaica Plain, MA 02130
1-800-669-8892 • email: ymaa@aol.com